AF601234

Laboratory Diagnosis and Clinical Biochemistry in Animals

The Authors

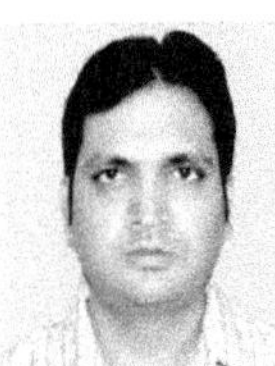

Dr. Rajesh Kumar Verma, born in Ambedkar Nagar district of Uttar Pradesh, graduated from the DUVASU, Mathura in the year 2010 and qualified his master's degree in Veterinary Microbiology from the College of Veterinary Science and Animal Husbandry, Narendra Deva University of Agriculture and Technology, Kumarganj, Faizabad in 2012. Dr. Verma was gold medallion in M.V.Sc. degree and cleared ICAR- NET. He published 10 research/clinical articles in different national and international journals of repute. Presently Dr. Verma is working as an Assistant Professor in the College of Veterinary Science and Animal Husbandry, Narendra Dev University of Agriculture and Technology, Kumarganj, Faizabad (U.P). He reorganized for reestablished the Clinical Laboratory in the Department of Teaching Veterinary Clinical Complex as per guidline of the Veterinary Council of India.

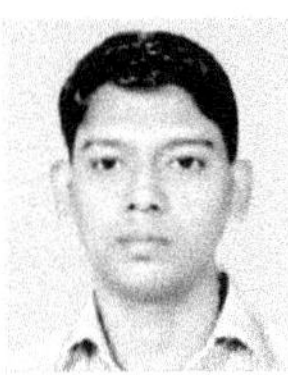

Dr. Awadhesh Prajapati, born in Gorakhpur district of Uttar Pradesh, graduated in Veterinary Science from DUVASU, Mathura in 2010. He completed M.V.Sc in Veterinary Bacteriology from Indian Veterinary Research Institute Izatnagar, a premier veterinary research institute in India. He was meritorious student during his graduate and post graduate program. He has cleared ICAR-JRF, ICAR-SRF, UGC- NET, and CSIR- NET. He has published more than 8 research papers and review articles in national and international journals of repute. Presently, he is working as Senior Technical Officer in biosafety laboratory of ICAR- National Institute of Veterinary Epidemiology and Disease Informatics, Bengaluru.

Laboratory Diagnosis and Clinical Biochemistry in Animals

Rajesh Kumar Verma

Awadhesh Prajapati

2016

Daya Publishing House®

A Division of

Astral International Pvt. Ltd.

New Delhi – 110 002

Cataloging in Publication Data--DK
Courtesy: D.K. Agencies (P) Ltd. <docinfo@dkagencies.com>

Verma, Rajesh Kumar, author.
Laboratory diagnosis and clinical biochemistry in animals / Rajesh Kumar Verma, Awadhesh Prajapati.
pages cm

ISBN 978-93-86071-11-8 (International Edition)

1. Veterinary clinical pathology. 2. Veterinary clinical biochemistry. I. Prajapati, Awadhesh, author. II. Title.

SF772.6.V47 2016 DDC 636.089607 23

Published by : **Daya Publishing House®**
A Division of
Astral International Pvt. Ltd.
– ISO 9001:2008 Certified Company –
4760-61/23, Ansari Road, Darya Ganj
New Delhi-110 002
Ph. 011-43549197, 23278134
E-mail: info@astralint.com
Website: www.astralint.com

Dedicated to beloved

Parents

Acknowledgements

We wish to put on record our sincere thanks to Dr. A.K. Gangwar, Associate Professor (Veterinary Surgery and Radiology), and Dr. Rajesh Kumar, Assistant Professor, (Animal Reproduction Veterinary Gynaecology and Obstetrics) for making valuable suggestions during preparation of manuscript.

We wish to express our heartfelt gratefulness to Dr. Rajesh Kumar Joshi, Professor and Head, Department of Microbiology and Dr. H. N. Singh, Dean College of Veterinary Science and Animal Husbandry for their valuable suggestion, constant encouragement.

The completion of this book would not have been possible without the continuous support of our family's members.

I express my indebtedness to my father Sri. R.S. Verma who had always been a constant source of inspiration, encouragement, and lamp in all the moment of depression, without him, this achievement was not possible. All the credit of my success goes to my respected mother Smt. Shobha Verma. She gave me proper guidance, good education, best advice from childhood that's how I am just here. I would like to thank our wife Rachana and son Tejas who have always been cooperative and helpful during the preparation of this book.

Rajesh Kumar Verma

Finally I extend my acknowledgements with gratitude, the support and love of my family- my parents Smt. Atvari Prajapati and Sri. Ramadhar Prajapati; brother like friend, Yogisharadhya and my wife, Indrasani. They all keep me going, and this book would not have been possible without them.

Awadhesh Prajapati

Preface

We have ventured to write this textbook with the hope to provide useful and specific information to undergraduate veterinary student according to Veterinary Council of India syllabus and to veterinarian engaged in diagnosis laboratory services. Since the beginning it has always been a challenge for the veterinarian to make efficient and timely diagnosis of animal disease which solely depends upon his professional expertise. Trained and skilled veterinarian in laboratory diagnosis is need of hour to increase the efficiency of treatments and to decrease indiscriminate use of antibiotic. An effort is made through this book to provide comprehensive knowledge of common diagnosis test useful to access the animal health condition.

This book has been prepared as per the VCI syllabus for the B.V.Sc & A.H. degree programme and is divided in 19 chapters which includes microbiological, parasitological, biochemical, pathological and toxicological techniques. All the procedure described in stepwise manner, which is easy to understood and performed in laboratory. An effort is made to provide more and latest information through the boxed segment in most of the chapters. In the last of book, a series of objective questions are included for the practice purpose which helps in boost the self confidence in students for their university exam.

Overall this book provides sufficient information regarding laboratory diagnosis of animal. Besides undergraduate students, it will also useful to the teachers, field veterinarians, scientists, postgraduate researchers and disease investigation workers in their day to day laboratory investigations. We hope that all this will ensure the continuing success of this textbook in the future.

Rajesh Kumar Verma

Awadhesh Prajapati

Contents

Abbreviations

AGPT: Agar Gel Precipitation Test
ALT: Alanine Amino-Transferase (ALT)
AST: Aspartate Aminotransferase
BGA: Brilliant Green Agar
BSC: Biosafety Cabinet
BSL: Biosafety Level
BSP: Bromsulphthalein
BUN: Blood Urea Nitrogen
CAMP: Christie, Atkins, And Munch- Petersen
CBPP: Contagious Bovine Pleuropneumonia
CCPP: Contagious Caprine Pleuropneumonia
CFT: Complement Fixation Test
CK: Creatine Kinase
CNS: Central Nervous System
CSF: Cerebrospinal Fluid
DLC: Differential Leucocyte Count
DM: Diabetes Mellitus
ELISA: Enzyme-Linked Immunosorbent Assay
EMB: Eosin Methylene Blue
EPG: Egg Per Gram
ESR: Erythrocyte Sedimentation Rate

FMD: Foot And Mouth Disease
FNAC: Fine-Needle Aspiration Cytology
GDH: Glutamate Dehydrogenase
GDV: Gastric Dilatation Volvulus
GFR: Glomerular Filtration Rate
GGT: Gamma-Glutamyl Transferase
GOD-POD: Glucose Oxidase - Peroxide
GT: Germ Tube Test
H&E: Hematoxylin and Eosin Stain
HA: Haemagglutination
HCl: Hydrochloric Acid
HDL: High-Density Lipoprotein
HEPA: High-Efficiency Particulate Arrestance/Air
HI: Hemagglutination-Inhibition
IMViC: Indole Test; Methyl Red Test; Voges-Proskauer Test, and Citrate Test.
KOH: Potassium Hydroxide
LCB: Lactophenol Cotton Blue
LDH: Lactate Dehydrogenase
LDL: Low-Density Lipoprotein
LFT: Liver Function Tests
MCH: Mean Corpuscular Hemoglobin
MCHC: Mean Corpuscular Hemoglobin Concentration
MCV: Mean Corpuscular Volume
MIC: Minimum Inhibitory Concentration
MLA: MacConkey Lactose Agar
MR: Methyl Red
NaCl: Sodium Chloride
ONPG: Ortho-Nitrophenyl Galactoside Test
PAS: Periodic Acid–Schiff
PCR: Polymerase Chain Reaction
PCV: Packed Cell Volume
PPR: Peste des Petits Ruminants
SAT: Slide Agglutination Test
SDH: Sorbitol Dehydrogenase

SGOT: Serum Glutamic Oxaloacetic Transaminase
SGPT: Serum Glutamic-Pyruvic Transaminase
TLC: Total Leukocyte Count
TSI: Triple Sugar Iron
USG: Urine Specific Gravity
VP: Voges–Proskauer
XLD: Xylose lysine deoxycholate agar

Chapter 1

Orientation to Veterinary Clinical Laboratory

Clinical Laboratory Orientation

Clinical laboratory involves the isolation, propagation and handling of pathogenic microorganisms that pose a risk to laboratory personnel and environments. The laboratory design must be such that the necessary precautions are taken to minimize the contaminants. Its design should be safe, pleasant and efficient to work.

There are mainly three types of disease diagnosis laboratories depending upon the types of investigations carried out.

1. **Clinical Pathology**: Hematology, Histopathology, Cytology, Routine Pathology.
2. **Clinical Microbiology**: Bacteriology, Virology, Mycology, Parasitology, Immunology, Serology.
3. **Clinical Biochemistry**: Biochemical analysis, Hormonal assays etc.

Layout of laboratory depends upon types services provided, the numbers and types of specimens that are processed. In a typical laboratory space is provided for each of the following:

- ☆ Sample receiving
- ☆ Sample storage and processing
- ☆ Open bench for routine work
- ☆ Staining and light microscopy
- ☆ Washing and Media preparation
- ☆ An isolation room for handling zoonotic organism

- Culture room
- Molecular diagnostic room
- Waste disposal
- Store room

Organization of Laboratory

Sample Receiving and Preparation Area

This area should be located near the laboratory entrance so that delivery man or other laboratory staffs need not to enter into the laboratory.

Open Bench

- Made up of non corrosive metal or stone, ease to cleaning and mopping.
- U-shaped modules or linear benches with appropriate sitting space which provide ease movement in laboratory.
- Provision of waste containers both for paper and biohazardous waste.
- Provision for storing completed cultures, stock cultures, reference books and teaching materials etc.

Bench Top/Work Top

- Should be made of materials that can be cleaned and disinfected easily, durable, easily repaired and stain resistant.
- Should be impervious to water and resistant to acids, alkalis, organic solvents and moderate heat.

Flooring and Ceiling

- Should be smooth, easily cleanable, impermeable to liquids and resistant to chemicals and disinfectants.

Instruments

- Microscopes (light, fluorescent, phase dark field)
- Centrifuges
- Dry heat oven
- Incubators (radiant heat, CO_2)
- Water baths
- Vortex mixer
- Anaerobe chamber
- Refrigerators, freezers, Ultra-low freezers
- Biological safety cabinet

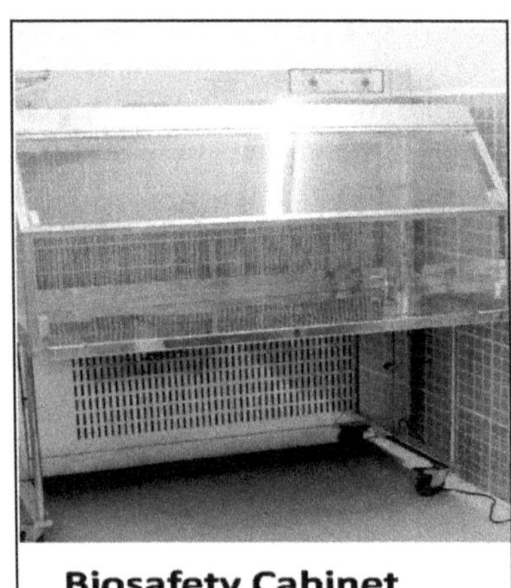

Biosafety Cabinet

Culture Room

- ☆ Bacteriology culture work and virological work should be done in separate culture room.
- ☆ Do not keep heavy instrument or machine in culture room. Place only essential items require for culture work.
- ☆ Strictly prohibit the entry of visitors.

Storage

- ☆ Storage space should be adequate since insufficient storage space makes hindrance in routine work area.
- ☆ Make provision of both Short term storage and Long term storage of item.

Safety and Security

- ☆ Keep fire extinguishers in the work area.
- ☆ Provision of eyewash stations, safety showers, sprinkler systems, fire alarms, spill control kits, emergency power and lighting.
- ☆ Easily approachable separate exit.

The following basic steps should be practice in the microbiology lab.

- ☆ Wear lab coat while working in the lab.
- ☆ Put your coat, books and other items in specific area locations.
- ☆ Keep doors and windows closed to prevent contamination.
- ☆ Personnel wash their hands after they handle viable materials and animals.
- ☆ Do not eat, drink and handle contact lenses or apply cosmetics in the laboratory.
- ☆ Mouth pipetting is prohibited. Use mechanical pipetting devices.
- ☆ Wipe the bench top/table with gauze pads saturated with 70 per cent ethanol or other suitable disinfectant at the beginning and end of the work.
- ☆ All contaminated materials (needles, cultures, glass wares, culture fluids and other contaminated liquid wastes) sterilize by proper method (autoclaved or disinfectant).
- ☆ Never put stationary item (pencil, labels etc.) in the mouth in the lab.
- ☆ Perform all procedures to minimize the creation of splashes or aerosols.
- ☆ Clean and disinfect the culture spilled area immediately.

Biosafety

The safety of personnel from infections who is working in a biological laboratory is called as biosafety. Different biosafety levels are required for handling different microorganisms safely and reduce or eliminate exposure to potentially hazardous agents. It can be achieved only through safety practices, safety methods, safety equipments, safe laboratories and biosafety cabinets etc. Four different biosafety levels are available for microbiological and biomedical laboratories for personnel and environmental protection based on the experiments they carry out.

Biosafety Level 1 (BSL 1)

- Suitable for work involving well-characterized agents of no known or of minimal potential hazard to laboratory personnel and the environment.
- Requires no special design laboratory.
- Work may be done on an open bench top, using gloves and some sort of facial protection.
- Basic microbiology laboratory practice employed for decontamination of surface.
- Lab materials used for cell and/or bacteria cultures are decontaminated by autoclave.

> **Types of Biosafety Cabinate (BSC)**
>
> **Class I biosafety cabinet** will provide personnel and environmental protection, but not product protection.
>
> **Class II biosafety cabinet** will provide personnel, environment and product protection.
>
> **The Class III biosafety cabinet** is a totally enclosed ventilated cabinet. Operations within the Class III cabinet are conducted through attached rubber gloves.

Agents

Bacillus subtulis, many strain *Escherichia coli* and *Staphylococcus* spp., Infectious Canine Hepatitis virus.

Biosafety Level 2 (BSL 2)

- Suitable for work involving agents of moderate potential hazard to personnel and the environment.
- These agents are hazardous through the ingestion and inoculation or contact with mucous membrane
- Biosafety cabinet and centrifuges with sealed rotors or safety cups are to be used along with appropriate personal protective equipment (i.e., gloves, laboratory coats, protective eyewear).
- Extreme precautions be taken in handling contaminated sharp items and wastes are decontaminated through autoclaves.

Agents

Influenza viruses types A, B, C other than notifiable avian influenza (NAI); Newcastle disease virus; Orf (parapox virus); *Campylobacter* spp.; *Chlamydophila psittaci* (nonavian); *Clostridium tetani; Clostridium botulinum; Corynebacterium* spp.; *Erysipelothrix rhusiopathiae; Haemophilus* spp.; *Leptospira* spp.; *Moraxella* spp.;

Pseudomonas spp.; *Salmonella* spp.; *Staphylococcus* spp.; *Yersinia enterocolitica; Yersinia pseudotuberculosis; Aspergillus fumigatus; Microsporum* spp.; *Trichophyton* spp.

Biosafety Level 3 (BSL 3)

- ✰ Suitable for work involving agents of highly potential hazard to personnel and the environment.
- ✰ These agents may be transmitted by the airborne route, often have a low infectious dose to produce effects and can cause serious or life-threatening disease.
- ✰ Specific training is required in handling these agents.
- ✰ Additional primary and secondary barriers are required to minimize the release of infectious organisms into the laboratory and the environment.
- ✰ A waste disposal system (effluent treatment plant) available within area.
- ✰ Air flow in laboratory through ducted air system only that draw clean air from outside and exhaust air discharged through HEPA filters.

Agents

Rabies virus; Equine encephalomyelitis virus (Eastern, Western and Venezuelan); Japanese B encephalitis virus; Louping ill virus: *Bacillus anthracis; Burkholderia mallei* (*Pseudomonas mallei*); *Brucella* spp.; *Chlamydia psittaci* (avian strains only); *Coxiella burnetti; Mycobacterium bovis.*

Biosafety Level 4 (BSL 4)

- ✰ Suitable for work with dangerous and exotic agents.
- ✰ These agents pose a high individual risk of aerosol-transmitted laboratory infections for which vaccines or other treatments are not available.
- ✰ Use of a Hazmat suit (positive pressure suite) and a self-contained oxygen supply is mandatory.
- ✰ Entrance and exit will contain multiple showers, a vacuum room, an ultraviolet light room, and other safety precautions designed to destroy all traces of the biohazards.
- ✰ Multiple airlocks system to regulate air pressure in laboratory.
- ✰ All incoming and outgoing air and water will undergo possible decontamination procedures.
- ✰ Laboratory staff should train in handling extremely hazardous infectious agents.

Agents

Smallpox virus, Ebola virus, Hemorrhagic fever viruses, Marburg virus, Lassa fever.

Practices in different Biosafety Level

Practices	*Agents*	*Primary Barriers*	*Secondary Barriers*
BSL-1	Not known to consistently cause diseases	None required	Open bench top, sink required.
BSL-2	Associated with human diseases and transmitted through per-cutaneous injury, mucous membrane ingestion route	Class I or II biosafety cabinets **PPE:** Lab coats, Gloves, Face protection.	Autoclave Eyewash
BSL-3	Associated with Human diseases. with potential for aerosol transmission	Class I or II biosafety cabinets **PPE:** Lab coats, Gloves, respiratory protection.	Double door access Negative airflow Filtration of exhaust air through HEPA
BSL-4	Life threatening disease, transmitted through aerosol route, no vaccine and medicine available	All procedures conducted in Class III bio safety cabinets or Class I/II bio safety cabinets in combination with full body, air supplied positive pressure suit	Isolated building decontamination system for liquid and solid waste

Collection, Preservation, Transport and Processing of Clinical Specimens

Collection of Samples

General precaution measure taken before collection of sample

- ☆ Minimize the contamination of sample collection.
- ☆ Sample should be representative of lesion and in proper amount.
- ☆ Sample should be sealed in sterile container and properly labeled with name, source, date and time of collection, brief history of diseases and clinical tentative diagnosis.
- ☆ Specific preservative should be used to prevent deterioration of sample if there is any delay in transportations.

Collection of Blood

Objective: To diagnose the existing disease condition, if any.

Requirements: Collection tubes, Sterilized syringes and needles, Sprit and 70 per cent ethanol, Cotton.

> The **gauge** of the needle refers to the outer diameter of the needle.
>
> Gauge numbers is inversely proportional to the outer diameters.
>
> **Common gauge needle used in different animals**
>
> Cattle and buffaloes: 16-18 G
>
> Sheep and goats: 18- 20 G
>
> Dogs: 20-22 G

Procedure

1. Blood collection prefer in early morning (12 hour after feeding).

2. Complete the requisition and label the tubes.
3. Select vein site and apply the pressure/tourniquet above it so that vein got engorged.
4. Clean the area.
5. Perform the vein puncture by needles and syringes.

Heparin accelerates the action antithrombin III which neutralizes thrombin and prevents conversion of fibrin form fibrinogen

EDTA prevents coagulation by chelating calcium.

Sodium fluoride inhibits the enzyme enolase and inhibits glycolysis.

Separation of Plasma

Blood plasma is prepared by spinning a tube of fresh blood containing an anti-coagulant (Citrated, EDTA or Heparinized) in a centrifuge for at least 15 minutes at 2000 to 3000g.

Serum

Blood serum is blood plasma without fibrinogen or the other clotting factors (*i.e.*, whole blood minus both the cells and the clotting factors).

Procedure

1. Collect the blood from animal without anticoagulant
2. Allow the blood to clot at room temperature
3. Centrifuge the tube for at least 10 minutes at a minimum speed of 1500g
4. Separate the straw color supernatant serum from clotted blood cells with the help of micro pipette/pasture pipette and place in a sterile tube
5. Store the tube at -80°C till further use.

Ammonium and potassium oxalate mixture also called as **Heller and Paul Mixture** is commonly used for anticoagulant.

Ration of potassium and ammonium oxalate must be **2:3** to keep the morphology of the RBCs.

Commonly Used Anticoagulants

Anticoagulant	*Amount (per 10 ml blood)*	*Advantage*
EDTA	10-20mg	For routine haematology
Heparin	1-2 mg (0.2 ml of 1 per cent solution)	Least effect on size and haemolysis of RBCs
Sodium oxalate	20 mg	Used mainly from prothrombin time test
Sodium citrate	10-20 mg	Used for blood transfusion
Sodium fluoride	100 mg	Na-F prevents glycolysis in RBCs by inhibiting the enzyme 'enolase'

Common Blood Collection Site in different Animals

Animals	*Site*
Cattle/Buffalo	Jugular vein
Horse	Jugular vein
Camel	Jugular vein
Sheep	Jugular vein
Goat	Jugular vein
Pig	Ear vein, Anterior venacava
Dog	Cephalic vein, Recurrent tarsal vein, Saphenous vein
Cat	Cephalic vein, Jugular vein
Poultry	Wing vein, heart
Rat	Retro-orbital plexus, cardiac puncture
Mice	Retro-orbital plexus, cardiac puncture (Terminal),Tail clipping, Saphenous vein
Rabbits	Cardiac (anesthetized only), marginal ear vein
Guinea pig	Cardiac (anesthetized only), anterior venacava/subclavian vein
Hamsters	Saphenous vein cardiac puncture
Rhesus monkey	Cephalic vein, Saphenous vein

Storage and Preservation of Blood and its Components

At room temp, blood can be kept up to 4 hours.

At 4°C, blood can be kept up to 24 hours.

At -20°C, blood can be kept up to 3 months.

Fresh Frozen Plasma (FFP) can be stored up to one year at -30°C or lower.

Cryopreservation of red blood cells is done in glycerol to store rare units, usually for up to 3 years.

It is necessary to maintain the cold chain at all times during transportation and storage.

Anticoagulant mechanism of CPD solution

Glucose - Provides ATP through glycolytic pathways.

Citrate - Prevents coagulation by chelating calcium.

Sodium di-phosphate - Maintain the pH

Addition of **adenine** improved preservation capability of CPD and prolonged the storage of blood/red cells at 2-4°C to 35 days.

Collection of Urine

Objective: For the diagnosis of renal disease, diabetes mellitus, presence of urinary calculi, jaundice, ascites, edema, haematuria, haemoglobinuria etc.

Material requires: Sterile polypropylene container, catheter, wax.

Different Methods for Collection of Urine Sample

Polythene bags: A polythene bag applies over the urethra and tie with the help of rope over the back. **(Method of choice in male)**

Stimulation of urethra: Massaging urethral opening through vulva in cattle, buffaloes, sheep and goat.

Pressure on urinary bladder: Applying pressure on urinary bladder through rectum in large animals.

Syringe and needle method: Used in small animals for direct and aseptic collection of urine from bladder.

Catheterization: A catheter is inserted into the bladder through vagina in female.

Metabolic cages: Used in laboratory animals (rat and mice) for urine collection.

Preservation

Urine samples should be examined immediately after collection or can be preserved by following methods.

Refrigeration at 4°C

Thymol @ 100mg/100 ml of urine (it may give false reaction for albumin).

Formalin @ 1 drop/10 ml of urine

Porphyrins and urobilinogen are light sensitive and so urine need to be collected into amber-coloured containers.

Boric acid is the most common preservative used for culture and sensitivity assay of urine.

Cells in urine can be fixed with ethanol (500 ml/l) but the addition of 20g/l PEG improves preservation.

Choice of Preservative for Analysis of Substances in Urine

Substance	*Preservatives*
Amylase, total protein and electrolytes	Refrigeration
Heavy metal	No preservative or only refrigeration
Calcium and phosphorus	Hydrochloric acid
Steroids and catecholamine metabolites	Glacial acetic acid
Uric acid, creatinine, amino acids, and a few steroids (estradiol).	Boric acid

Collection of Faeces

Objective: Indication of jaundice, hepatitis, anemia, presence of blood in faeces etc.

Methods

Large animal: Faeces can be collected directly from rectum or from ground when freshly voided.

Small animals: Generally faecal swab is used.

After collection sample should be immediately placed in a sterile container and dispatched to laboratory at 4°C (ice pack) in a transport medium.

Preservation

- ☆ Refrigeration at 4°C
- ☆ 10 per cent Formalin.

Collection of Milk

Objective: For the laboratory diagnosis of mastitis and other udder infection.

Procedure

1. Clean the udder with water and 1:100 solution of $KMnO_4$.
2. Clean the hands of collecting person with soap and antiseptics.
3. Discard first few drops of milk to avoid debris.
4. Collect 5-10 ml of milk for testing.

Collection of Synovial Fluid

Objective: For the diagnosis of arthritis and other joint diseases.

Procedure

1. Anaesthetize with local anesthesia.
2. Collect the synovial fluid from affected joints with an 18 gauze needle.
3. Apply wound adhesive to prevent infection.
4. Amount of synovial fluid
   Cattle/buffalo/horse/camel (large animals): **5-10 ml**
   Dog/cat/sheep/goat (small animal): **0.5- 1.0 ml**

Preservation: 3.8 per cent sodium citrate (0.1 ml/ml of synovial fluid)

Collection of Cerebrospinal Fluid (CSF)

Objective: Diagnosis of CNS disorders.

Site of Collection

Sub occipital region: Horses, Sheep, Goats, Pigs and Dog

Lumbosacral region: Cattle and buffaloes

Procedure

1. Anesthetize the animal.
2. Insert a 12 cm long needle with stylet in the mid line of soft depression between the dorsal process of lumbar vertebrae and the anterior end of median sacral crest, the point at the level of line joining anterior border of tuber coxae.
3. Removed the stylet and collect the CSF by syringe.

Collection of Ascitic Fluid and Hydatid Cyst Fluid

Ascitic Fluid

Abdominal Paracentesis Procedure

1. With the help of 70 per cent alcohol disinfect the abdominal surface.
2. Use 18-22 gauze sterile needles to remove ascites fluid.
3. Allow the ascites fluid to drip from the needle into a sterile collection tube.
4. Allow to stand at room temperature for 30 min.

Preservation: Storage at – 70°C.

Cyst Fluid

1. Aspirate by sterile needle in aseptic conditions.
2. Centrifuge at 1000 rpm for 5 min, take the supernatant.

Preservation: Storage at -20°C.

Common Preservation Methods for different Clinical Samples

Sample	*Preservatives*
Serum	Sodium azide (0.1 per cent) or methiolate (0.01 per cent)
Milk	Refrigeration at 4ºC.
	5 per cent boric acid in one tenth of total milk volume
Urine sample	Refrigeration at 4ºC
	Thymol @ 100mg/100 ml of urine (it may give false reaction for albumin).
	Formalin @1 drop/10 ml of urine
Faeces	Refrigeration at 4ºC
	10 per cent Formalin
Histopathological samples	10 per cent formalin
Synovial fluid	3.8 per cent sodium citrate (0.1 ml/ml of synovial fluid)
Cerebrospinal fluid	Sodium fluoride for estimation of glucose.
	Other examinations no need to add any preservative.

Transport Medium and its Composition

Stuart Transport Medium

Composition

Thioglycolic acid	2 ml
Sodium hydroxide	12-15 ml

Aqueous Calcium chloride	20 per cent
Distilled water	900 ml

Mix all the ingredients; add 1N sodium hydroxide solution and finally adjust pH to 7.2.

Buffered Glycerol Saline

Composition

Glycerol	300ml
Sodium chloride	4.2 g
Disodium Hydrogen phosphate	10.0 g
$Na_2 H PO_4$ Anhydrous	15.0 g
Phenol red (aq 0.02 per cent)	15.0 ml
Distilled Water	700 ml

Process

1. Dissolve NaCl in distilled water and add glycerol in this solution.
2. Add disodium hydrogen phosphate to dissolve.
3. Add phenol red indicator and adjust pH to 8.4.
4. Distribute the 6 ml solution in universal containers (screw- capped bottles of 30 ml capacity).
5. Autoclave the containers at 121°C for 15 minutes.

Charcoal Transport Medium

Composition

Sodium Chloride	4.00g
Potassium chloride	0.20 g
Dipotassium phosphate	1.70 g
Charcoal	10.0 g
Agar	4.00 g

Mix the ingredients in 1000 ml of Distilled water, adjust pH to 7.2 and kept this container in autoclave at 121°C for 15 minutes.

Dispatch of Specimens

- ✰ Specimen send to the nearby laboratory with minimum deterioration and to minimize the hazards must be primary concern.
- ✰ If any delay is expected before the specimen is processed, it is generally preferable to freeze the specimen at -70°C in a thermo flask or thermo cool box for avoiding adverse environmental condition.

- ☆ The specimens must be secured (without any leak or break) and packed before dispatch with proper labeling.
- ☆ It is always better to get the consent of the laboratory and permit from authority before sending any specimen for processing.
- ☆ The permit or license should be placed in an envelope and pasted on outside of the parcel.
- ☆ Information and case history should always accompany the samples in water proof plastic envelop along with container.

Important Information's Required along with Clinical Sample

Name and address of owner.

Telephone and fax number of owner.

Senders name, postal, telephone, fax, E-mail address.

Diagnostic test requested for suspected disease.

Species, breed, age, sex and identity of animal.

Date of sample collection and submission.

List of samples submitted and transported.

History of the condition like clinical signs observed duration, treatment given and vaccination status etc.

Requisition slip for laboratory examination of clinical specimens

Date .... **Case No.** ....

Name of address of owner

....

....

....

Animal species .... **Breed** .... **Sex** .... **Age** ....

History/ Symptom/ Treatment, if any

....

....

....

Clinical specimen: faeces/ tissue/ serum/ blood/ urine/ synovial fluid/ milk/ skin scrapping/ others

....

....

Examination requested

....

Signature of forwarding clinician

Chapter 2

Clinical Significance and Interpretation of Serum Glucose, Protein, Lipid, Ketone Bodies, Minerals, Electrolytes, Bilirubin, Creatinine, Blood Urea Nitrogen (BUN), and Uric Acid from Samples

Serum Glucose

The most frequently for diagnosis of disturbance in carbohydrate metabolism glucose level is determined in the blood.

The Main Disturbances of Carbohydrate Metabolism are Hypoglycemia and Hyperglycemia

Hyperglycemia

This can be vary in severity from the mild hyperglycemia occurring after a meal, exercise, stress or corticosteroid treatment to very extreme hyperglycemia found in uncontrolled diabetes mellitus.

Diabetes Mellitus

This is common condition in both cat and dog and is unusual in ruminant. Based on the human medicine classified into 2 type:

1. **Type 1 DM (insulin dependent)**: Most common factor is auto antibodies which react against with beta cell of pancreas. It is uncommon in animals other than the dog and occurs more commonly in younger animals. Ketoacidosis is common manifestation.

2. **Type 2 DM (non insulin dependent)**: It occurs when insulin secretion is not enough to maintain the blood glucose level or body cell (Fat, liver, and muscle cells) do not respond correctly to insulin. It trend to occur in older animal and often associated with obesity.

Clinical Biochemical Finding in Diabetes Mellitus

1. Large amounts of glucose in urine.
2. Large volume of urine and increased frequency of micturition (Polyuria)
3. Eats more frequently (Polyphagia).
4. Increase in free fatty acid level in blood and liver.
5. Increased ketone bodies in blood and urine (ketonemia and ketonuria).
6. Increased catabolism of tissue protein, loss of weigh and increased formation of urea.

Sample Collection in DM

a) **Fasting blood Sugar (FBS)**: The blood sample is collected after the patients (animal) fasts for 12 hours or overnight.

b) **Post-Prandial Blood Sugar (P P B S)**: After the patient (animal) fasts for 12 hours, a meal is given which contains starch and sugar (approx. 100 g). Blood is collected 2 hours after the ingestion of the meal.

c) **Random Sample**: Blood is collected any time without prior food restriction.

Blood is usually collected from a vein and kept in a bottle containing sodium fluoride (NaF) and potassium oxalate mixed at proportion of 1: 3. Usually 4 mg of the mixture is required. Both the substances act as anticoagulant and Na F prevents glycolysis in RBC's by inhibiting the enzyme 'enolase'.

Oral Glucose Tolerance Test (OGTT)

Glucose Tolerance is defined as the capacity of the body to tolerate an extra load of glucose. It is used mainly to diagnose diabetes. An oral glucose tolerance test is a series of blood glucose measurements taken after you drink a sweet liquid that contains glucose. Normally the blood glucose level remains relatively constant.

Procedure

1. A blood sample will be collected when the subject arrives after 8-12 hour fasting.
2. Estimate the plasma glucose level in collected blood. This is the fasting blood glucose value which is baseline for comparing other glucose values.
3. Dissolved 75 g of glucose in 300 ml of water (for children 1.75 g/kg body weight up to a maximum of 75 g). Let the patient drink it within 5 minutes.
4. Collect blood samples at timed intervals of 1, 1.5 2, 2.5 and 3 hours after drinking the glucose.

Interpretations

Normal Response: Fasting blood sugar is normal. After 1 hour level rises, but remain below the renal threshold of 180 mg/dl. It returns to normal fasting level within 2 hours.

Diabetic Curve: Fasting level of 140 mg/dl and 2 hour venous blood glucose of 200 mg/dl or more are diagnostic of diabetic condition.

GOD - POD Method

Principle

Glucose is oxidized by glucose oxidase (GOD) and produce gluconate and hydrogen peroxide. The hydrogen peroxide is then oxidatively coupled with 4 amino- antipyrene (4-AAP) and phenol in the presence of peroxidase (POD) to yield a red quinoeimine dye that is measured at 505 nm. The intensity of colour is proportional to concentration of glucose in the sample.

$$\text{Glucose} + 2H_2O + O_2 \xrightarrow{(GOD)} \text{Gluconate} + H_2O_2$$

$$2H_2O_2 + \text{4-AAP} + \text{Phenol} \xrightarrow{(POD)} \text{Quinoeimine Dye}$$

Absorbance of the colored solution is directly proportional to the glucose concentration when measured at 505nm.

Reagent

Glucose Oxidase	20000 µ/l
Peroxidase	1200 µ/l
4-AAP	0.246 mmol/l
Glucose Standard	100 mg/dl

Procedure

1. One reagent blank and one standard are sufficient for each assay series.
2. Adjust the instrument to zero with distilled water.
3. Pipette into a cuvette as fallow

Particulars	*Blank*	*Standard*	*Sample*
Reagent 1	1000µl	1000µl	1000µl
Dist. Water	10µl	–	–
Reagent 2	–	10µl	–
Sample	–	–	10µl

4. Mix well and incubate for 15 min at room temperature or 7 min at 37°C. Measure the absorbance of standard and sample against reagent blank at 505 nm.

Calculation

Glucose concentration in the sample can be calculated using the following formula:

Glucose (mg/dl) = Absorbance of Sample/Absorbance of Standard X Conc. of Std. (mg/dl)

Conversion factor: mg/dl x 0.0555= mmol/l.

Complications of DM

Early

1. Diabetic Ketoacidosis
2. Comas: Ketoacidotic, lactacidotic, hyperosmolar non-ketotic, hypoglycaemic.

Late

1. **Microangiopathy**: Neuropathy, nephropathy, retinopathy.
2. **Macroangiopathy**: Coronary heart disease, cerebrovascular diseases, peripheral angiopathy.

Hypoglycemia

Blood glucose falls below the normal level. Commonly associated with over dosing of insulin in treatment of diabetes mellitus

Other condition associated with hypoglycemia

- Hypothyroidism- Cretinism, myxodema
- Insulin secreting tumor of pancreas
- Hypoadrenalism (Addison's disease)
- Hypopituitarism
- Severe exercise
- Starvation

Reference Ranges of Serum Glucose (mg/dl) in different Animal

Animal	*Serum Glucose (mg/dl)*
Cows	40 – 75
Sheep	45 – 80
Goats	50 – 75
Dog	75 – 120
Horse	60 – 120
Pig	70 – 120

Serum Protein

Serum contains a large variety of proteins. More than hundred different proteins have been identified so far. Albumin and the various globulins constitute the bulk of the total amount of proteins present in serum. Biuret method is most widely used for estimation of protein in serum.

Biuret Method

Principle

Cupric ions form chelates with the peptide bonds of proteins in an alkaline medium. Sodium potassium tartrate keeps the cupric ions in solution. The intensity of the violet colour that is formed is proportional to the number of peptide bonds which, in turn, depends upon the amount of proteins in the sample.

Reagents

Biuret Reagent – 3 mg of copper sulphate is dissolved in 500 ml of water. 9 g of sodium potassium tartrate and 5 g of potassium iodide are added and dissolved. 24 g of sodium hydroxide, dissolved separately in 100 ml of water is added. The volume is made up to 1 litre with water. The reagent is stored in a well-stoppered polythene bottle.

Biuret blank – This is prepared in the same way as the biuret reagent with the difference that copper sulphate is not added.

Standard protein solution – A 6 g/100 ml solution of bovine albumin in water prepared and used as standard.

Procedure

1. Label 3 test tubes as 'Unknown', 'Standard' and 'Blank',
2. Put 5 ml of biuret reagent into each tube.
3. Add 0.1 ml of serum into 'Unknown', 0.1 ml of standard protein solution into 'Standard' and 0.1 ml of water into 'Blank'.
4. Mix and allow standing for 30 minutes.
5. Read 'Unknown' and 'Standard' against 'Blank' at 540 nm or using a green filter.

Calculations: Serum total proteins (g/100 ml) = Avg U/Avg S x 6

Interpretations

- ☆ The normal range of serum total proteins is 6-8g/100ml in all species.
- ☆ An increase in serum total proteins occurs in dehydration due to haemoconcentration.
- ☆ An increase may also see in multiple myeloma, macroglobulinaemia, chronic infections, chronic liver disease and autoimmune disease and autoimmune diseases.

- A decrease in serum total proteins may results from heavy losses of proteins in urine as in nephritic syndrome, protein malnutrition, intestinal malabsorption and protein losing enteropathy.
- A decrease may also see in shock, burns, crush injuries, haemorrhage, un-treated diabetes mellitus etc.

Serum Albumin, Globulin and A: G Ratio

Clinical Significance and Interpretations

- The normal range of serum albumin is 2.5–5.5 g/100 ml and serum globulin ranges from 2–6 g/100 ml. The A: G ratio is roughly 2:1 through it may range from 1.2: 1 to 2.5:1.
- A low A/G ratio may reflect overproduction of globulins or under production of albumin or selective loss of albumin from the circulation. A high A/G ratio suggests under production of immunoglobulin.
- Decrease in serum albumin may occur in protein under nutrition, intestinal malabsorption, and protein losing enteropathy, liver disease, wasting diseases, nephritic syndrome and haemodilution.
- A severe decrease may see in nephritic syndrome, haemodilution and albuminaemia an autosomal recessive genetic disease.
- Serum globulin may decrease in shock, burns, and haemorrhage etc.
- Serum globulin increases in multiple myeloma, macroglobulinaemia, chronic liver disease, chronic infections and autoimmune diseases.

Serum Lipid Profile

Lipid profile is a group of tests that are often ordered together to determine heart disease risk. It includes total cholesterol (TC), low-density lipoprotein cholesterol (LDL-C), high-density lipoprotein cholesterol (HDL-C) and triglyceride (TG).

Triglycerides

Most triglycerides are found in adipose (fat) tissue. During exercises/work some triglycerides circulate in the blood and provide fuel to muscles. Triglycerides increase in blood after meal when fat is being sent from the gut to adipose tissue for storage. The test for triglycerides should be done when you are fasting and no extra triglycerides from a recent meal are present. Normal plasma triglycerides concentration is around 1 mmol/lit in dog and 0.4 mmol/lit in horse. When triglycerides are very high there is a risk of developing pancreatitis.

Interpretations

Hypertriglyceridemia: Hypothyroidism, Diabetes mellitus, Starvation, Hyper-adrenocorticism, Biliary obstruction, Pancreatitis, Glomerulopathy, Hepatic lipidosis, Acromegally, Obesity, Anti thyroid therapy, Primary lipoproteinaemias, Hyperchylomicronaemia, equine hyperlipidaemia.

Cholesterol

Cholesterol is an essential substance of body. It forms cell membranes, tissue, hormones that are essential for development, growth and reproduction, and acids that are needed to absorb nutrients from food. A small amount of the body's cholesterol circulates in the blood in complex particles called lipoproteins. The level of serum cholesterol is influenced by fat rich diet of animal containing saturated fatty acids. Estimation of cholesterol level in blood is indicative of liver and thyroid function.

Cholesterol Levels

Normal plasma concentration about 7-8 mmol/lit in dog, 5-6 mmol/lit in cat and 2-3 mmol/lit in herbivores. Cholesterol level has only diagnostic important in canines and felines. In herbivore the level are usually very small and increases are not specifically associated with particular condition.

Interpretations

Hypercholesterolemia: Nephritic syndrome, Hypothyroidism, Stress, High fat Diet, Bile duct obstruction, Leukemia, Pregnancy.

Hypocholesterolemia: Hyperthyroidism, Anaemia, Hepatic disease, Intestinal obstruction, polycythemia.

High Density Lipoproteins Cholesterol (Good Cholesterol)

The main function of high density lipoproteins (HDL) is the transfer of cholesterol from peripheral tissues to the liver. HDL particles are mostly synthesized in the liver, and a minor part in intestinal cells. The nascent HDL particles contain phospholipids, cholesterol, ApoE and Apo A, and are discoid in shape. In the circulation, they assume a spherical shape due to the acceptance of ApoC and free cholesterol from other lipoproteins and non-fatty cells.

Interpretations

Determination of HDL-cholesterol is used in prevention diagnosis. Blood concentration of HDL- cholesterol is related with the occurrence of atherosclerotic disease, primarily coronary heart disease (CHD) and peripheral circulation impairments. The lower blood concentration of HDL-cholesterol, the greater the risk of the disease.

Low Density Lipoproteins-Cholesterol (Bad Cholesterol)

LDH is a type of lipoprotein that carries cholesterol in the blood. It is considered undesirable because it deposits excess cholesterol in tissues and organs as well as walls of blood vessel and contributes to hardening of the arteries and heart disease. LDL cholesterol testing is an important part of a CDH prevention strategy. It is used to further assess the risk of CDH when total cholesterol and/or HDL cholesterol results are abnormal. LDL cholesterol is used to monitor patients with prior CDH, other atherosclerotic disease, or diabetes mellitus.

Serum Ketone Bodies

Ketone bodies (Acetone, Acetoacetic acid and β-hydrobutyric acid) are intermediary products of fat metabolism and their presence in the blood and then in the urine are indications that the metabolism is disordered or incomplete. Normal plasma β-hydrobutyric acid concentration under 1 mmol/l and it is often under detectable. Increase in level associated with metabolic acidosis. This occurs in poorly controlled diabetes mellitus and also in starvation.

Ketosis of varying intensity may occur in all mammalian species and can be brought forth, for example, by starvation, low carbohydrate and high fat diets, cold exposure, anesthesia, impaired liver function, hypoglycemia, and endocrine disorders such as diabetes or growth hormone and other endocrine excesses. Females of any species are more susceptible to ketosis than corresponding males, and this predisposition is exaggerated during lactation or pregnancy. Ketosis occurs in animal mainly in two situations

Diabetic ketoacidosis: Most common in DM I where insulin activities almost zero virtually cell fail to utilize any glucose in spite of high glucose level in blood. This situation often accompanies diabetic coma and hyperkalemia.

Absolute carbohydrate deficiency: This is most commonly seen in cattle and sheep with acetonaemia and pregnancy toxaemia and usually associated with hypoglycemia.

Serum Minerals

Calcium

Calcium is an essential mineral which is involved in many body systems. These include the skeleton, enzyme activation, muscle metabolism, blood coagulation and osmoregulation. In the blood calcium exists as 50 per cent ionized, 40 per cent protein bound and 10 per cent complexes with anions such as citrate and phosphate. Only ionized calcium is biologically active in bone formation, neuromuscular activity, cellular biochemical processes and blood coagulation. Factors governing the total plasma concentration are complex and include interaction with other chemical moieties, proteins and hormones. Calcium, phosphorus and albumin metabolism are interdependent.

Interpretations

Serum calcium level varies from 8-11mg/100 ml in healthy animals.

Elevated levels (Hypercalcaemia): Lymphoproliferative disease (dogs), Hypoadrenocorticism (dogs), Malignant neoplasia, Primary renal failure (CRF or Familial), Primary hyper-parathyroidism, Hypervitaminosis D.

Low level (Hypocalcaemia): Hypoalbuminae, Malabsorption, Acute pancreatitis, Renal secondary hyperparathyroidism, Eclampsia, Primary hypoparathyroidism, Post thyroidectomy (cats), Nutritional secondary hyperparathyroidism, Ethylene glycol poisoning, Acute renal failure (especially post renal obstruction), Glucocorticoid therapy.

Phosphorus (Inorganic Phosphate)

Phosphorus is present in blood as inorganic phosphate and in combination with several organic compounds including carbohydrates, lipids and nucleotides. Inorganic phosphorus is present mainly in serum. Serum phosphorus is primarily regulated by the kidney through the action of parathyroid hormone. Abnormal levels are caused by variations in dietary intake, decreased renal excretion and the hormonal imbalances that affect serum calcium.

Interpretations

The normal range of serum inorganic phosphorus is 4.0–8.0 mg/100 ml in adult animals.

Elevated levels: Prerenal, renal and post renal azotemia, Hyperthyroidism, Hyper-parathyroidism, Primary Hypoparathyroidism, Tissue necrosis, Osseous Neoplasia, Hypervitaminosis D.

Low levels: Malignant neoplasia, Osteomalacia, Glucocorticoid therapy, Oral phosphate-binding agents, Hyperadrenocorticism, Hypovitaminosis D, Renal tubular defects.

Serum Electrolytes

Sodium

Sodium is predominantly extracellular due to the sodium pump mechanism. Renal function is the single most important homeostatic mechanism in relation to the plasma concentrations of sodium and potassium.

Slight hyponatraemia is common in small animals. Marked hyponatraemia or sodium: potassium ratio $< 27:1$ indicates further investigation. Marked hyponatraemia may cause fluid movement into cells with an effective on neurological function. Hypernatraemia is uncommon in small animals. It almost always indicates water intake which is inadequate to balance fluid losses. Marked Hypernatraemia may lead to neurological signs due to the net movement of water out of the cells.

Sodium levels reflect the relative amounts of water and electrolytes in the extra-cellular fluid. It is the principle determinant of ECF volume. Hyponatraemia occurs more commonly due to excessive losses than to reduced intake. Hypernatraemia indicates water loss in excess of electrolytes.

Interpretations

Elevated levels (Hypernatraemia): Diabetes mellitus, Diabetes insipidus, Hyper-adrenocorticism, Increased sodium intake, Moderate dehydration, Pyometra, High protein diets Osmotic cathartics, Extreme exercise, Drug therapy (*e.g.* corticosteroids).

Low level (Hyponatraemia): Hypoadrenocorticism, Severe dehydration (vomiting and diarrhoea), Diabetes mellitus, Ruptured urinary tract, Administration of low sodium fluids, End stage chronic renal failure, Diuretic therapy, Psychogenic polydipsia, Acute renal failure (polyuric phase), Hypertension (congestive heart failure), Hypoalbuminaemia, Drug therapy (*e.g.* NSAID's).

Potassium

Plasma potassium levels are not always a good indicator of intracellular levels. In acidosis condition exchange of H^+ and K^+ ions leads to the depletion of intracellular potassium and elevated plasma potassium. The converse occurs in alkalosis. Hypokalaemia may lead to neurological, muscular and cardiac signs. In most cases, hyperkalaemia arises due to a diminished ability to excrete potassium. Marked hyperkalaemia is potentially life threatening causing bradycardia and cardiac arrest.

Interpretations

Elevated level (Hyperkalaemia): Acute renal failure Hypoadrenocorticism, Massive tissue damage, Metabolic acidosis (*e.g.* liver failure) Low sodium intake, Urethral obstruction, Drug action (*e.g.* digitalis), Bladder rupture.

Low level (Hypokalaemia) Diuretic therapy, Diabetes mellitus Polyuric disorders, Vomiting and diarrhea, Chronic renal failure (particularly cats), Insulin therapy, Hypomagnesaemia Chronic hepatic disease Thrombocytosis, Steroid administration, Chronic renal failure (terminal event), Excessive bicarbonate therapy, Excessive mineralocorticoid therapy, Hyper-adrenocorticism, Acute renal failure (poly uric phase), Fanconi's syndrome, Hypothermia, Alkalosis (respiratory or metabolic).

Chloride

Chloride is present in highest concentrations in the ECF and tends to accompany sodium movement by passive diffusion.

Interpretations

Elevated levels (Hyperchloraemia): Dehydration, Acidosis, Respiratory alkalosis.

Low levels (Hypochloraemia): Gastro-intestinal loss (high bowl obstruction), Low salt diet Respiratory acidosis.

Serum Bilirubin

Bilirubin is an endogenous anion derived mainly (85 per cent) from destruction of senescent RBCs by reticuloendothelial cells in spleen and 15 per cent from the other haemoproteins (mainly hepatic cytochromes). Porphyrin ring of hemoglobin breaks in to biliverdin, iron and goblin. Biliverdin forms bilirubin in presence of biliverdin reductase. This bilirubin is now carried to the plasma where it is loosely bound to albumin and α-1 globulin and this form of bilirubin is termed as free bilirubin. In the liver this bilirubin is conjugate with glucuronic acid in presence of enzyme Glucuronyl transferase. Now it is known as conjugate bilirubin. Conjugate bilirubin is excreted in to biliary canaliculi by the hepatocyte and reaches in to small intestine with the help of biliary system. Bacterial flora of small intestine converts bilirubin to urobilinogen (reduced bilirubin). Some part of urobilinogen is excreted through faeces here by oxidized to urobilin which gives orange colour to faeces. Some part of urobilinogen reabsorbed by portal blood system goes to kidney and liver. Kidney removes it as urinary urobilinogen and in liver it is removed by hepatocyte and excreted into bile, thus completing the enterohepatic circulation of bile pigment.

Interpretations

Total bilirubin: This is measured as the amount, which reacts in 30 minutes after addition of alcohol. Normal range is 0.2-0.9 mg/dl (2-15μmol/l).

Direct Bilirubin: This is the water-soluble fraction. This is measured by the reaction with diazotized sulphanilic acid in 1 minute and this gives estimation of conjugated bilirubin. Normal range 0.3mg/dl (5.1μmol/l).

Indirect bilirubin: This fraction is calculated by the difference of the total and direct bilirubin and is a measure of unconjugated fraction of bilirubin.

Serum Creatinine

Creatinine like urea is a by-product of muscle energy metabolism that filtered from the blood by the kidneys and excreted into the urine. Production of creatinine depends on an individual's muscle mass, which usually fluctuates very little. With normal kidney function the amount of creatinine in the blood remains relatively constant and normal. Its measurement provides an indirect assessment of the **glomerulas filtration rate (GFR)**. Creatinine is very little affected by liver function so an elevated blood creatinine is a more sensitive indication of impaired kidney function than the Blood Urea Nitrogen.

Interpretation in Elevated Levels

Renal, pre renal and post renal azotaemia, Severe prolonged excretion or exercise, Acute myositis or muscle trauma, Cooked meat diet, Pituitary hyperactivity, New born foals- may be a normal feature or may indicate birth hypoxia or Placental dysfunction.

Blood Urea Nitrogen (BUN)

BUN is a waste product produced from the breakdown of protein. Blood urea is removed from the body via the urine, so BUN levels increase as kidney function decreases. Any increase in protein introduced into the intestines to be digested (such as a very high protein diet of meat or blood proteins from a bleeding ulcer) can increase BUN in the blood. Dehydration also increases the BUN value. BUN is measured as a simple blood test.

Urea	= BUN X 2.14
Mol. Wt. of Urea	= 60
Urea Nitrogen	= 28
Factor = 60/28	= 2.14

Interpretations

Elevated levels: Renal azotaemia, Acute renal failure, Shock, Chronic renal failure, High protein diet, Fever, Reduced cardiac output, Hyperthyroidism (cats), Hypoadrenocorticism, Gastrointestinal haemorrhage, Prolonged exercise, Corticosteroid therapy, Post renal Azotaemia, Feline urological syndrome, Bladder rupture, Calculi, Neoplasia, Perineal hernia, Prostatic enlargement.

Low levels: Polydipsia/polyuria, Hepatic insufficiency, Protein malnutrition, Over hydration, Late pregnancy, Anabolic steroids.

Bun: Creatinine Ratio

A BUN test may be done with a blood creatinine test. Blood urea nitrogen (BUN) and creatinine tests can be used together to find the BUN to creatinine ratio (BUN: creatinine).

Interpretations

BUN-to-creatinine ratio varies between 10:1–20:1

High ratio: Sudden (acute) kidney failure or blockage in the urinary tract (such as a kidney stone), bleeding in the digestive tract or respiratory tract.

Low ratio: Low protein diet, Severe muscle injury

Uric Acid

Purines such as adenosine and guanine from the breakdown of ingested nucleic acids or from tissue destruction are converted into uric acid mainly in the liver and then transported by the plasma to the kidney where it is filtered by glomerulus.

Interpretations

Increased levels of uric acid are associated with gout, renal failure and large dietary intake of purines.

Chapter 3

Clinical Significance and Interpretation of Urine Examination

Urine Analysis

Urine Analysis is very useful indicator and can provide much valuable information in regard to urinary system as well as other organs or system in body like carbohydrate metabolism, kidney and liver function and acid-base balance.

Renal disease- Proteinuria, blood cells (RBCs and WBCs), abnormal specific gravity and casts

Urinary bladder infection- Presence of bacteria, proteinuria and leukocytes

Hepatic disease- Bilirubinuria, altered urobilinogen

Diabetes mellitus- Glycosuria and ketonuria

Diabetes insipidus- low specific gravity of urine and when water is with held from urine, failure to concentrate urine

Neoplasm- Neoplastic cells

Haemolysis- Haemoglobinuria and level of urobilinogen increased

Acidosis and alkalosis

Collection of Urine

- ☆ Container of urine collection should be clean and sterile. It should be made up of either glass vial or disposable plastic.
- ☆ Dark coloured glass contain should be used to prevent the certain constituents like bilirubin and urobilinogen from sunlight if immediate examination is not possible.
- ☆ Best time for urine collection is early morning likely to contain constituents of diagnostic significance.

- Before collection of urine first stream of urine should be left, it contains leukocytes, cellular debris, exudates from urethra, genital tract and prepuce.
- A fresh sample of urine should be examined as soon as possible otherwise important constituents may be degrade for example urea split into ammonia and urine become alkaline.
- If immediate analysis is not possible then urine preservation is necessary.
- Refrigeration of urine at 4°C - 2 to 3 hr.

Preservatives- Thymol, Toluene, formalin, chloroform and boric acid.

Urinalysis

There is three method of urine analysis

A. Physical examination

B. Chemical examination

C. Microscopic examination

A. Physical Examination of Urine

Volume of Urine

The amount of volume produced per day depends upon various factor like diet, fluid intake, climate, exercise, size and body weight. Urine volume is inversely proportional to specific gravity except in diabetes mellitus (glycosuria increases both volume and specific gravity).

Normal Volume of Urine in Different Animal

Animals	*Urine (liter/day)*
Cattle	9.0- 23 (14.5)
Horse	2-11 (4.7)
Dog	0.5 to 2.0 (1.0)
Pig	2.0-6.0
Goat/Sheep	0.5 to 2.0 (1.0)

Polyuria (Increased volume of urine)

Causes- Nephritis, Diabetes mellitus, Pyometra and hepatic disease.

Oligouria (Decreased volume of urine)

Causes- Shock, fever, acute renal failure and heart disease

Colour of Urine

Normal urine is typically transparent and yellow coloure by the presence of urochrome pigment. The intensity of color is in part related to the volume of urine collect and concentration of urine produced. Abnormal urine colour may be due to presence of endogenous or exogenous pigments.

Amber urine: Conjugated bilirubin

Red urine: Haemoglobin (blood, free), myoglobin, porphyria, drugs (phenolphthalein, deferoxamine, some phenothiazines).

Smoky/brown urine: Altered blood (acid hematin), alkaptonuria (turns brown on standing), melanin (*i.e.*, disseminated melanoma)

Dark orange urine: Drugs (pyridium, rifampin, others)

Fluorescent yellow: Vitamins

Foamy urine: Proteinuria, conjugated bilirubin

Turbid/cloudy urine: WBC's, urates, phosphates

Fat globules on surface: Fat embolization

Odour

The normal odour of urine is due to presence of volatile organic acids. The urine of males of porcine, feline and caprine has strong odour. An ammonical odour emanates free decomposed urine due to urea breakdown. The presence of ketone bodies produces a sweetish and fruity odor and detected in association with pregnancy toxaemia, acetonaemia and diabetes mellitus. Excretion of certain drugs gives characteristic odour. Abnormal foul odour denotes excessive urine breakdown by bacteria as seen in cystitis or when the urine is stored too long in a container at room temperature.

Turbidity

Urine is typically clear but may become less transparent with pigmenturia, crystalluria, haematuria, pyuria, lipiduria or when other compounds such as mucus are present. Depending on the cause, increased turbidity may disappear with centrifugation of the sample.

Specific Gravity

Specific gravity is measure of relative amounts of solids in solution (urine). It is measured by urinometer. The urine is filled in cylinder and urinometer is left in the urine which should not touch the wall of cylinder.

Interpretation of urine specific gravity (USG) depends on the clinical presentation and serum chemistry findings. Dehydrated animal have higher specific gravity urine (hypersthenuric) than normal range. Dilute urine in a dehydrated or azotemic animal is abnormal and could be caused by renal failure, hypo- or Hyperadrenocorticism, hypercalcemia, diabetes mellitus, diuretic therapy, hyperthyroidism or diabetes insipidus. Glucosuria increases the refractive index of urine, resulting in an increased USG despite increased urine volume.

Specific Gravity of Urine in different Animal

Species	Range	Average
Cattle	1.025- 1.045	1.035
Sheep/goat	1.015- 1.045	1.030
Horse	1.020- 1.050	1.030
Dog	1.015- 1.045	1.025
Cat	1.020- 1.040	1.030

B. Chemical Examination

Urine pH

Urine pH is typically acidic in dogs and cats (**6.0-7.0**) and alkaline in horses (**8.0**) and ruminants (**7.4- 8.4**), but varies on diet, medications, or presence of disease.

Increased pH - urinary tract infects by urease containing bacteria (*e.g. Staphylococcus, Proteus*), Alkaluria

Decreased pH- Metabolic acidosis, Renal tubular acidosis, Hypokalaemia

Protein

Normally protein is not found in the urine. Once urine filtered at glomerulus, proteins are almost completely reabsorbed in the proximal tubule. Proteinuria, therefore, can be the result of increased filtration at the glomerulus or decreased tubular reabsorption.

Glomerular Proteinuria is associated with the presence of larger molecular weight protein losses. The nephritic syndrome is associated with very large losses of protein. Tubular Proteinuria is associated with smaller amounts (of lower molecular weight protein molecules). Small losses of protein in urine can be seen with vigorous exercise and pregnancy.

Sulphosalicylic Acid Test

Principle: Sulphosalicylic acid precipitate urine proteins.

Procedure

1. Take about 2.0 ml of Sulphosalicylic acid in a test tube.
2. Add urine drop by drop so that the two layers remain separate.
3. Appearance of a white precipitation ring at the junction of two layers shows the presence of protein.
4. When the two layers are, mixed, whole solution becomes turbid, which confirm protein in the urine.

Heller's Ring Test

Principle: Strong acid precipitate urine proteins.

Procedure

1. Take 3.0 ml of conc. HNO_3 (nitric acid) in a test tube.
2. Add 3.0 ml of urine in such a way that two fluids do not mix.
3. Appearance of white ring indicates the presence of protein.

Indications

Renal diseases (*i.e* nephritic syndrome, nephritic syndrome, tubular disease, urinary tract infections and tumors).

Glucose

Glucose is the predominant sugar in urine. Temporary elevation of glucose excretion can occur after treatment with some drugs, shock and during pregnancy. Repeated positive testing is almost always diagnostic for diabetes.

Benedict's Test

Principle

Glucose is a reducing sugar which reduces cupric ion (Cu^{++}) to cuprous ion (Cu+) in Benedict's reagent. Cuprous is less soluble and forms cuprous oxide and produces different colours *i.e.* green, orange, yellow or red depending on the amount of sugar present.

Procedure

1. Take 5.0 ml of Benedict's reagent in a test tube.
2. Add few drops (8 to 10 drops) of the urine.
3. The solution is then boiled vigorously and then allowed to cool.
4. Green, orange, yellow or red precipitate means the presence of sugar whereas if sugar is absent, there will not be any colour change.

Colour Change	*Percentage of Sugar*
Green	Less than 0.5
Orange	More than 0.5 and less than 1.5
Yellow	1.5
Red	More than 2.0

Interpretations

Diabetes mellitus, Excessive endogenous or exogenous Glucocorticoid, Stress, Proximal renal tubular defect (such as primary renal glucosuria).

Ketones (Acetone, Acetoacetic acid and beta-hydroxybutyric acid)

Ketones are spilled into urine when the body cannot utilize glucose (as in diabetes) and metabolize fatty acids. This catabolism is incomplete, resulting in the formation of large amounts of ketone bodies.

Rothera's Test

Principle: Nitroprusside reacts with acetoacitic acid in the presence of ammonium hydroxide and ammonium sulphate to give permanganate colour.

Procedure

1. Saturate 5 ml of urine with ammonium sulphate.
2. Add 2-3 drops of concentrated ammonium hydroxide and a few drops of freshly prepared 5 per cent solution of sodium nitroprusside and shake.
3. A positive test is indicated by development of a permanganate tinge which gradually deepens.

Interpretations

Primary ketosis (ruminants), Diabetes mellitus (small animals), Prolonged fasting or starvation.

Bile Pigment

Bilirubin is formed by the degradation of heme. Normally it is not excreted into urine. Only the conjugated form of bilirubin, often termed direct bilirubin, is excreted into urine in pathological condtions.

Gmelin test

Principle

Nitric acid oxidizes the yellow coloured compound *i.e.* bilirubin to biliverdin (green), bilicynin (blue), bilifusin (brown), choletelin (yellow) etc.

Procedure

1. Take about 3.0 ml of conc. nitric acid in a test tube.
2. Add equal volume of urine in such a way that two fluids do not mix.
3. At the point of contact note various coloured rings, green, red and reddish tallow.

Interpretations

Liver diseases, Viral hepatitis, Haemolytic, Bile ducts obstruction

Bile Salt

Sulphur Flower Test

Principle: Bile salts reduce surface tension of fluids in which they are present.

Procedure

1. Cool 10.0 ml of urine in a test tube to 17°C or lower
2. Sprinkle a little sulphur powder on the surface of urine.

3. The presence of bile acid is indicated if the sulphur sinks to the bottom of the urine.

Clinical significance and interpretation same as bile pigment

Blood

Red coloure urine is indicative of haemorrhage (hematuria), intravascular hemolysis (haemoglobinuria), or myoglobinuria. A positive result should be interpreted with microscopic examination of urine sediment

Benzidene Test

Principle

Haemoglobin acts as a peroxidase enzyme and converts Benzidine powder in to a coloured compound. In presence of H_2O_2 giving dirty blue or green precipitate which on standing turns brown.

Procedure

1. Add 2.0 ml of urine in 3.0 ml of saturated solution of Benzidene in glacial acetic acid.
2. Add 1.0 ml of hydrogen peroxide.
3. A blue or green indicates a positive test.

Interpretations

Haematuria (intact erythrocytes incorporated in the urine): Glomerulonephritis, Stones, Tumors, TB, Coagulopathy, Infection, Vasculitis, Schistosomiasis, Leptospirosis.

Haemoglobinuria (Haemoglobin in urine due to excessive haemolysis of RBCs): Haemoglobinuria, Baccilary haemoglobinuria, Leptospirosis, Babesiasis, Haemolyic disease of new born, Burn, Chemicals poisoning like Sulphonamide, Mercury and Copper and plants (Brooms, Hellebore, Savin, Colchicum etc.).

Myoglobinuria: Azoturia-Paralytic Equine Myohaemoglobinuria (Black to brown colour urine, and differentiated from hematuria by absence of intact erythrocytes in the urine sediments).

C. Microscopic Examination

Procedure for Preparation and Analysis of Urine Sample

1. Take fresh urine or warmed previously refrigerated urine in a conical centrifuge.
2. Centrifuged it gently (1,000 rpm for 5 minutes) and decant the supernatant and mixed the sediment by gently tapping the tube or pipetting up and down.
3. A drop of sediment is placed on a clean glass slide and a cover slip is placed on it avoiding air bubbles.

4. Place the slide on microscope stage and see under low power (10X objective).
5. The presence of crystal is reported at this magnification as 1+, 2+, 3+, or light, moderate, heavy. Identification of crystal type should be attempted.
6. Now change to high power (40X) and rescan the area. The number of erythrocytes, leucocytes and epithelial cells, casts, crystals and bacteria seen per high power field are counted and recorded. It is advisable to count in 5-10 different fields and then average the numbers unless there are very large numbers seen.
7. For further identification of cells types or to differentiate bacteria from particles the 100X oil emersion objective can be used.
8. Brownian motion of particles can usually be distinguished from motile bacteria at 100X power.

Normally sediments are classed two broad seagents

A. **Organized:** Erythrocytes, Leucocytes, Microorganism, Epithelial cell, Parasites, Spermatozoa.

B. **Unorganized sediment:** Fat globules, Precipitated crystals, Acidic, Alkaline.

Urinary exosomes contain apical membrane and intracellular fluid and are normally secreted into the urine from all nephron segments. These may carry protein markers of renal dysfunction and structural injury.

A. Organized Sediments

Erythrocytes

- Hemorrhage in genitourinary system.
- If the blood comes during onset of urination the source of haemorrhage is urethra.
- The bladder haemorrhage is characterized by blood mixed last portion of urine, while urine is mixed with blood in kidney haemorrhage.
- Haemorrhage also occurs as a result of catheterization, bladder puncture and manipulation of bladder.

Leucocytes

- Ten or more WBC/mm3 of urine indicate urinary tract infection.
- Pyuria, Inflammation, Infection, Trauma or Neoplasia, Catherization

Epithelial Cells

In normal urine sample epithelial cells are present in very low in number. Squamous epithelial cells in urine come from urethra, bladder and vagina. These are the largest cells in sediment and have small round nucleus. The epithelial cells of renal tubules are smaller, round or polyhedral in shape and these are larger than leucocytes.

The number of epithelial cells increases in cystitis or other inflammatory condition of urinary passage.

Microorganism

Bacteria: Cystitis, Pyelonephritis (Identified by Gram's staining).

Yeast: Colourless, round to avoid bodies with double refractile walls.

Fungi: Distinct segmented fungal hyphae in urine.

Parasites: The ova of the following parasites may be seen in urine sediment.

Stephanurus dentatus- (Swine kidney worm), *Dioctophyma renale*- (Giant kidney worm of dog and mink), *Capillaria plica*- (bladder worm of dog, cat and fox) *Dirofilaria immitis.*

Protozoa: Protozoa generally nor present in urine. Sometimes Trichomonads and Giardia are found in urine as contaminants of genital tract.

Spermatozoa: Easily recognizable by their shape and common in the urine of male.

Cylindruria (Casts)

Casts are elongated; cylindrical bodies appeared in the sediment of urine. These structures formed in the lumen of renal by mucoprotein congealing and may contain cells.

Hyaline casts: Mucoproteineous, colourless, semitransparent cylindrical structures with parallel side present in fever, exercise, circulatory disturbances and renal disease.

Epithelial Cellular Casts

- Formed from desquamated cells entrapment of sloughed tubular epithelial cells in the mucoprotein
- Observed in renal disease like degeneration of tubular epithelium and acute nephritis

Granular Casts

- Fine or course granules derived from degeneration of tubular epithelial cells.
- Typically have sharp borders with broken ends.
- Present in severe type of renal disease, necrosis of tubular cells.

Erythrocyte Casts

- Homogenous cylindrical mass, deep yellow or orange in colour.
- Renal haemorrhage and glomerulitis.

WBC Casts

- ☆ Leukocytes adhere to hyaline matrix.
- ☆ Renal tubules inflammation, pyelonephritis and kidney abscess.

Fatty Casts

- ☆ Numerous fat globules, colourless, when stained with Sudan III stain give orange to red colour.
- ☆ Disorders of lipid metabolism, such as diabetes mellitus.

Crystals

The presence of crystals in urine depends on the pH, the solubility and concentration of the crystalloid and colloids.

Normal acidic urine may contain amorphous urates and uric acid and less commonly calcium oxalate and hippuric acids.

Alkaline urine contains Triple and amorphous phosphate, calcium carbonate (especially in the urine of horse) and rarely ammonium urate crystal may be present.

The abnormal crystals in urine are minor significance except when urolithiasis is seen due to disturbance in protein metabolism and may result in cystine calculi.

Fat

- ☆ Round and highly retractile bodies of varying sizes.
- ☆ Stain orange to red with Sudan III stain.
- ☆ Indicative of fatty metamorphosis of the renal tubules, rupture of lymphatic's, obesity, diabetes mellitus, hypothyroidism, high fat diet or may be originate from extraneous source such as lubricated catheter or a greasy container.

Urine Examination Report

Date ____________________ **Case no.** ____________________

Name and address of the owner:

____

____

Species: ____________ **Breed:** ____________ **Sex:** __________ **Age:** __________

History/symptom/treatment, if any:

____

____

____

Physical and chemical examination	**Microscopic examination**
Colour: ______________________	**Leukocytes:** ______________________
Transparency: ______________________	**Erythrocytes:** ______________________
Odour: ______________________	**Epithelial cells:** ______________________
	______________________
Foam: ______________________	
Specific gravity: ______________________	**Casts:** ______________________
Reaction (pH): ______________________	**Crystals:**
	______________________
Protein: ______________________	**Microorganism:** ______________________
Glucose: ______________________	**Parasites:**
	______________________
Ketone bodies: ______________________	
Bile pigments: ______________________	

Pathologist:

Chapter 4

Evaluation of Acid-Base Balance and Interpretation

Acid and Bases

- The substance that generates H^+ in solutions (proton donor) is Acid. eg- HCl, H_2SO_4, CH_3COOH etc.
- The substances that accepts H^+ in solutions (proton acceptor) and are also substances that generate OH^- is base. *e.g.*, NH_4OH.
- Normal pH of blood is 7.4.
- Condition of too low pH of blood is acidemia (less than 7.35) whereas too high is alkalemia (more than 7.45).
- Abnormal physiological processes and pathological conditions disturb the acid base balance of the plasma.
- Most of the volatile acid is produced as CO_2 in cell respiration and is subject to the reaction:

  $CO_2 + H_2O \leftrightarrow H_2CO_3 \leftrightarrow H^+ + HCO_3^-$

Acid-Base Balance Regulation Mechanisms

Respiratory Regulation

- By increasing or decreasing rate of respiration to eliminate CO_2.
- In the normal subject control mechanisms insure the maintenance of adequate oxygen supplies and keep pCO_2 value in the region of 40+/- 5 mmHg.
- Drops to less than 70 mmHg, pO_2 give an effective stimulus to ventilation.

Renal Regulation

- Kidney maintain the ions balance of body through excretion of acid, retention of extant bicarbonates and production of new bicarbonates to replace that consumed in the buffering of nonvolatile acids.
- Increase of plasma bicarbonate leads to the production of new bicarbonates by the excretion of protons into urinary buffer systems.
- The protons are eliminated trough the formation of ammonium and the conversion of HPO_4^{2-} to $H_2PO_4^-$.
- High hydrogen ion concentration stimulates the secretion of hydrogen ions, leading to an increase of ammonium ion concentration.
- High pCO_2 stimulates the renal re-absorption of bicarbonate while low pCO_2 has the opposite effect.

Buffer System of Animal Body

1. Carbonic acid and Bicarbonate Ratio (1:20)
2. Monosodium phosphate: Disodium phosphate system
3. Plasma protein system
4. Oxyhaemoglobin: reduced haemoglobin system

Types of Acid Base Disturbances

1. Metabolic
2. Respiratory

Laboratory Marker of Acid-Base Disturbance

1. The arterial blood pH, pCO_2 and HCO_3
2. The anion gap

Metabolic Acidosis (↓pH↓HCO_3^-)

Decrease in bicarbonate concentration in body lead to metabolic acidosis condition. It occurs when large amount of carbonic acid is formed with the help of hydrogen ion and bicarbonate ion.

$$H^+ + HCO_3^- \longrightarrow H_2CO_3$$

Classified into Two Classes

1. High anion gap metabolic acidosis (HAGMA)
2. Normal anion gap metabolic acidosis (*i.e.* hyperchloraemic acidosis)

Compensatory Mechanism

Through lungs: Balance the ratio of carbonic acid and bicarbonate ion removal of CO_2 occurs through hyperactive breathing (hyperpnoea).

Through kidney: Conservation of bicarbonate ions by excretion hydrogen ions and non bicarbonate anions.

Laboratory Finding

- ☆ pH of Arterial blood < 7.35
- ☆ pH of Urine more acidic than normal (Arterial blood H+ > 44 nmol/l)
- ☆ Bicarbonate in plasma below than normal (Arterial blood HCO_3^- < 18 mmol/l)
- ☆ Chloride in plasma usually low
- ☆ Arterial blood pCO_2 < 35 mmHg (4.7 kPa)

Interpretations

Diarrhoea: Loss of bicarbonate ions from intestine.

Metabolic Ketosis: Ketone acids accumulate in tissues.

Renal disease: Retain organic acid

Acidic drugs: (Salicylate, Paracetamol toxicity), NH4Cl, NaCl etc.

Shock

Metabolic Alkalosis (↑pH↑HCO_3^-)

Increase in bicarbonate ions concentration in body lead to metabolic acidosis condition.

$$H_2CO_3 \longrightarrow H^+ + HCO_3^-$$

Clinical Signs

- ☆ Slow and shallow breathing.
- ☆ CNS excitability, tetany and convulsion.

Compensatory Mechanism of Body

Through lungs: To balance the ratio of carbonic acid and bicarbonate ion lungs hold CO_2 by slow breathing.

Through kidney: Kidney excretes bicarbonate ions by retaining hydrogen ions and non bicarbonate anions.

Laboratory Finding

- ☆ pH of Blood > 7.35 (H+ < 36 nmol/L),
- ☆ pH of urine more alkaline than normal
- ☆ Plasma bicarbonate level more than normal (HCO_3^- > 32 mmol/l)
- ☆ Plasma chloride and potassium level usually low
- ☆ Arterial blood pCO_2 > 45 mmHg (6.0 kPa)

Interpretations

- Excessive loss of acid through vomiting.
- Loss of potassium ion through X ray, over activity of pituitary, adrenal tumor and excessive use of corticosteroid drugs.

Respiratory Acidosis (↓pH↑pCO_2)

This arises from an acute or chronic excess of carbon dioxide, and depends on the rate of production as well as excretion of carbon dioxide.

Clinical Signs

- Respiratory embarrassment
- CNS depression through disorientation and coma

Compensatory Mechanism of Body

Bicarbonate ions are conserved by kidney by removing hydrogen ions and non bicarbonate anions.

Laboratory Findings

- pH of Blood: > 7.35
- pH of Urine more acidic than normal
- Bicarbonate in plasma higher than normal
- Chloride in plasma usually low

Interpretations

Pneumonia, Emphysema, Respiratory muscle paralysis, Pneumothrox, Barbiturate, Morphine poisoning *etc.*

Respiratory Alkalosis (↑pH↓pCO_2)

Respiratory alkalosis occurs when the respiratory system eliminates too much CO_2 from body that lead to reduction in H^+ generation. The decreasing H^+ concentration raises the blood pH above 7.45.

Clinical Signs

Rapid breathing, sometime tetany and convulsion.

Compensatory Mechanism of Body

Bicarbonate ions are removed by kidney by retaining hydrogen ions and non bicarbonate anions.

Laboratory Findings

- pH of Blood < 7.35
- pH of Urine more alkaline than normal

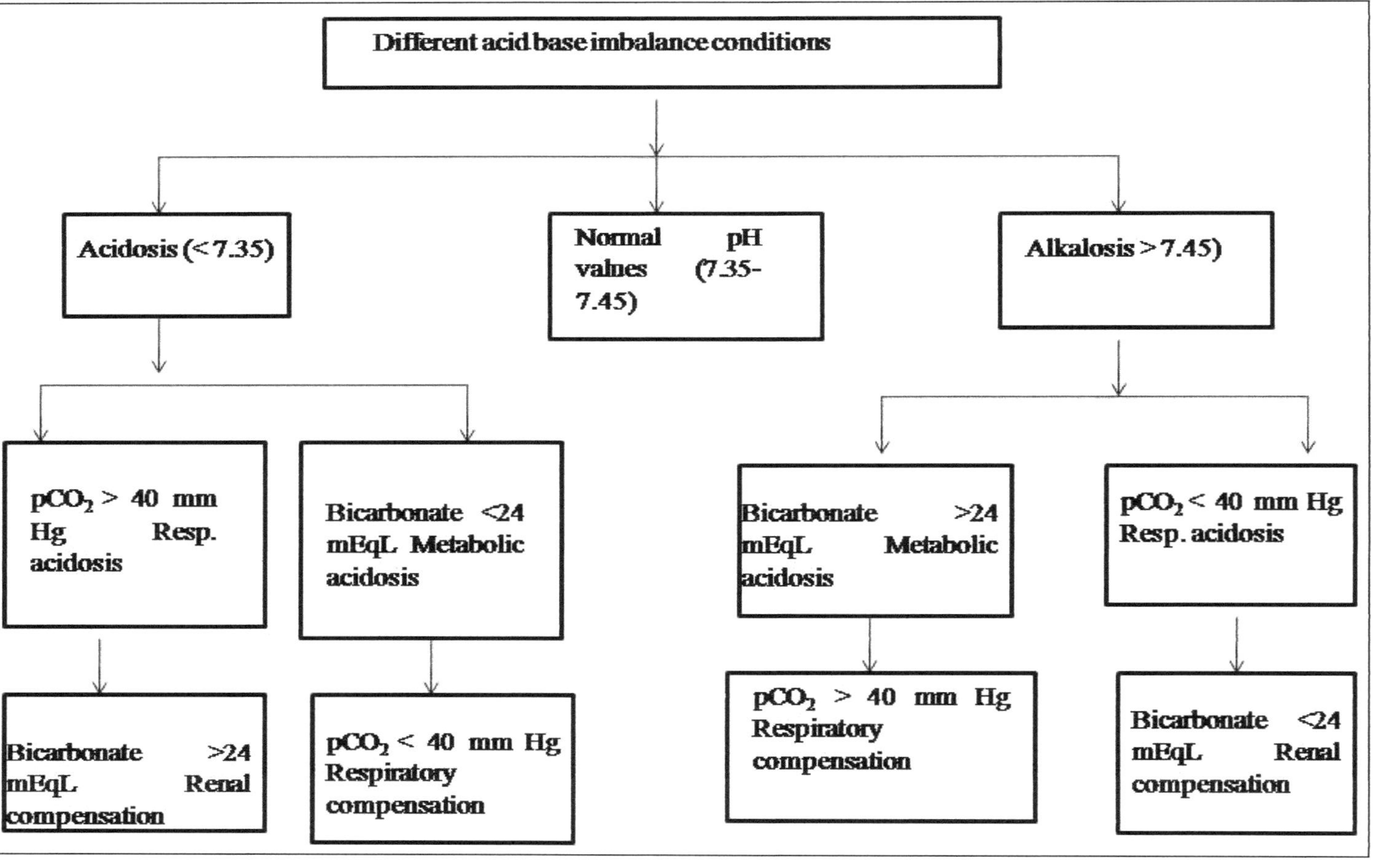

Flow Diagram of different Acid-Base Imbalance Conditions.

- ☆ Bicarbonate in plasma below than normal
- ☆ Chloride in plasma usually normal sometime may be high

Interpretations

Fever, Lack of Oxygen, Hysteria and Anxiety *etc.*

Chapter 5

Biochemical Aspect of Digestive Disorders and Endocrine Functions

Digestion is the process of breakdown of food into smaller components that can be more easily absorbed and assimilated by the body to build and nourish cells and provide energy. Digestive tract is made up of many organs like mouth, esophagus, stomach, small intestine, large intestine. Large intestine is made up of colon, rectum, and anus. Mucosa of mouth, stomach, and small intestine, contains small glands that produce juices for digest the food. The liver and the pancreas, produce digestive juices that reach the intestine through ducts. Digestive juices of liver stores in the gallbladder until needed in the intestine. Parts of the nervous and circulatory systems also play major roles in the digestive system. Animal should be treated by veterinarian when blood in stool, change in bowel habit, and severe abdominal pain like symptom is seen in animal by owner.

Disorder in Rumen Function

Many species of bacteria and other microbes involves in digestive process. They ferment proteins and carbohydrates in to small fatty acid chain, which are the energy sources for ruminants.

Acute Rumen Indigestion

High concentrations of lactic acid accumulate in the rumen and subsequently in the blood, when the animals consuming roughages are overloaded with readily fermentable carbohydrates. Due to fermentation of carbohydrates by bacteria present in rumen mixture of lactic acid is produced in which L-lactic acid is absorbed and metabolized but D- lactate cannot be utilized, which contributes to the acid load and cause metabolic acidosis. In the rumen the pH reduces to 5 or less due to accumulation of lactic acid, which allows the growth of acid producing bacteria. The osmolality of the rumen increases due to accumulation of lactate, which results in the absorption of water from the systemic circulation. Severe dehydration occurs in animal, which in turn may lead to hypovolemic shock.

Bloat

Bloat is a form of indigestion marked by excessive accumulation of gas in the rumen. During the rumen fermentation by microbes the gases (CO_2, methane) produced are removed by the process called eructation. Any obstruction in this process leads to accumulations of gases in rumen. Two general types of bloats are Simple bloat (Free gas) and Frothy bloat (Foamy). Simple bloat may occur in obstruction in passage of gas or increase production of gas in rumen while feeding of leguminous fodder or whole grain is predisposing for frothy bloat.

Urea Poisoning

When urea is fed at more than 3 per cent level Urea poisoning occurs in animals. Urea is hydrolyzed to CO_2 and NH_3 by urease enzyme. More ammonia formation occurs in animal body if excess urea is given to animal in his diet. The free ammonia crosses the cell membrane thereby producing harmful effects.

Rumen Function Test

Collect the rumen fluid from affected animal. It should be keep at room temperature for 9 hours before examination.

Gross examination

Color: Color of the rumen content fluid depends up on the type of the feed. The color should be from green to live to brownish green.

It will be green in grazing animals and grey in those animals that feed fodder betts, yellow brown in those that feed on silage or straw. Abnormally it may be greenish black in decomposition

Consistency: It is slightly viscous under normal condition. This viscosity is pronounced if large amount of saliva is included under the condition; it is advisable to discard the first part of the rumen fluid. It will be watery in case of acidosis and foamy in foamy bloat.

Odor: Under normal condition the odor of the rumen is aromatic odor and non replant

- Penetrating odor in acidosis
- Foul smelling in decomposition
- Different smell in active rumen

Total Acidity

The pH of the rumen fluid varies from 5.5 – 7 which may be affected by saliva which contains bicarbonate. The PH of rumen fluid will be alkaline in active rumen during starvation and urea poisoning, the bacteria responsible for digestion and production of acid are weak and alkaline is predominates. Urea poisoning, because of the breakdown of urea and formation of ammonia, the content of rumen becomes alkaline.

Indicator or Dip Stick Test

Insert an indicator/deep stick in to the fluid and observe the color change.

Titrable Acidity Test

Procedure

1. Pour 0.1N NaOH in the blurrette, write down the volume of the solution.
2. Measure 10ml of rumen content in the beaker and add 1-2 drops of phenophtaline indicator and mix well.
3. Let 0.1N NaOH be in the beaker drop to neutralize and go on until fresh color fluid comes out.

Result

Multiply total amount of NaOH by 10 *i.e.,* NaOH /ml 10 clinical units under normal condition the clinical units near 8 units but in abnormal conditions it could be 10–70 units.

Sedimentation Activity Time

Procedure

1. Directly use rumen fluid or filter the fluid allow to stand for a few minutes
2. The fine particles and infusoria settle down while floatation flows due to the production of gas by micro flora of rumen.
3. The time required for the setting down of infusoria and fine particles and floating of the production of gas by the microorganisms is known as the sedimentation activity time.
4. Under normal condition the SAT will be very weak floatation, slow or absent due to the absent of active microorganism, example in starvation.
5. In acidosis Lactobaccili are very active and there is large amount of gas production and floatation are very quick and large.

Bacteria Examination

To determine the dominate bacteria in the ruminal fluid.

Method: Gram stain

Lactic acidosis

No of Gram positive bacteria (*Streptococcus bovis*) increases.

Gram-negative bacteria is decreased or absent.

Number of ciliate protozoa decreased.

Procedure

1. Take a rumen fluid on the slide and make a smear
2. Dry and stain with gram stain
3. Observe under oil immersion for the presence or absence of the microorganisms. The bacteria in the rumen is referred as leading bacteria

Observation

- Observe Gram negative and Gram positive bacteria, write the dominate and the ratio
- Under normal condition gram negative bacteria are the dominate
- In the rumen of the animals feed on roughage, the large streptococci kidney shaped cocci, saracia are predominantly present
- Under acidosis condition Gram positive bacteria predominantly present

Microscopic Examination of Rumen Content Protozoan's

There are two form of protozoa to be predominate in rumen fluid, **Ciliates and Flagellates**. The ciliates are important because massive in numbers than the flagellates. There are 10–20 millions species which inhibits in the rumen as far as the physiological significance of these protozoan are considered to be not use full. However they are important in stabilizing bacterial digestive process.

Procedure

1. Take one or two drops of rumen fluid on the slide
2. Cover with cover slip and warm around 13 C
3. Observe under microscope
4. Grade the number of protozoa

Result

Abundant	+ + +
Moderate	+ +
Few	+
No protozoa	–ve

Interpretation

The size of the protozoa could be large or small and medium. There is no digestion in the rumen in the death of protozoa. Therefore, observe the proportion of death to alive one, in case of acidosis, No digestion *i.e.*, no protozoa.

Cellulose Digestion Test

Procedure

1. Take 10ml of rumen content in the test tube
2. Add about 0.3ml of 10 per cent glucose solution
3. Suspend cotton thread to the solution and incubate in 37 C for 48 hrs
4. The expected result is the action of microflora on the thread

Result

If the rumen is active, there will be break down of the thread.

Digestive Disorders in Non Ruminants

Vomiting

Vomiting is rapid, forceful ejection of gastric contents through the mouth due to a complex reflex act. There are many conditions for stimulation of vomiting like pyloric stenosis, intussusceptions, presence of parasites, presence of foreign objects, neoplasia, chronic gastritis, and presence of poisons. The loss of water and HCl occurs in vomiting. It causes dehydration and metabolic alkalosis with increased level of bicarbonate ion and decreased level of chloride ion concentration. Hypokalemia is another condition in vomiting due to increased urinary excretion during alkalosis. In severe vomiting renal tubular damage and kidney failure may occur due to potassium deficiency and hypovolemic due to dehydration.

Diarrhoea

Diarrhoea is a condition of rapid elimination of watery fecal material with increased frequency and volume or both. It may occur of any parasite, bacteria or viral infection in the intestinal tract, feeding poor quality diet, sudden dietary change, and food poisoning. Dehydration cause haemoconcentration, which leads to hypovolemic shock, this is characterized by decreased excretion of hydrogen, over production of lactic acid, hyperkalemia, and hypoglycemia.

Gastric Dilatation Volvulus (GDV)

Gastric dilatation volvulus (also known as twisted stomach, gastric torsion and GDV) is a medical condition in which the stomach becomes overstretched and rotated by excessive gas and fluid content causing mechanical and functional disturbances to pyloric out flow. Gastric dilatation volvulus in dogs is likely caused by a multitude of factors, but in all cases the immediate prerequisite is a dysfunction of the sphincter between the oesophagous and stomach and an obstruction of outflow through the pylorus. The increased pressure and size of the stomach may have several severe consequences, including:

1. Prevention of adequate blood return to the heart from the abdomen
2. Loss of blood flow to the lining of the stomach
3. Rupture of the stomach wall
4. Pressure on the diaphragm preventing the lungs from adequately expanding leading to decreased ability to maintain normal breathing.
5. Rotation of stomach can lead to blockage in the blood supply to the spleen and the stomach.
6. Shock and death of animal.

Lactose Intolerance

Lactose Intolerance means the body cannot easily digest lactose due to deficiency of enzyme lactase secreted by the intestinal cells. Lactose is a type of natural sugar found in milk and dairy products. In order for lactose to be absorbed from the intestine and into the body, it must first be split into glucose and galactose.

The glucose and galactose are then absorbed by the cells lining the small intestine. The enzyme that splits lactose into glucose and galactose is called lactase, and it is located on the surface of the cells lining the small intestine. Lactose intolerance is caused by reduced or absent activity of lactase that prevents the splitting of lactose (lactase deficiency). Lactase deficiency may occur for one of three reasons, congenital, secondary or developmental. Diarrhea, gas, and abdominal pain can occur when there is not enough lactase to digest milk products. Bovine neonatal diarrhea is also a indication of lactose intolerance. Nausea, vomiting, abdominal distension, cramps, flatulence, flatus, diarrhea and abdominal pain are clinical symptoms of lactose intolerance

Jaundice

Jaundice is a yellowish pigmentation of the skin, the conjuctival membranes over the sclerae (whites of the eyes), and other mucous membranes caused by high blood bilirubin levels. Bilirubin is a by-product of the daily natural breakdown and destruction of red blood cells in the body. The haemoglobin molecule that is released into the blood by this process is split, with the heme portion undergoing a chemical conversion to bilirubin. Normally, the liver metabolizes and excretes the bilirubin in the form of bile. However, if there is a disruption in this normal metabolism and/ or production and excretion of bilirubin, jaundice may result.

Endocrine Gland Disorder

Pancreatitis

Pancreas is major endocrine associated with digestive function. The primary diseases of the pancreas are pancreatitis. Pancreatitis is an inflammation of the pancreas. It usually presents with abdominal pain and can cause nausea and vomiting. This may be classified as acute pancreatitis or chronic pancreatitis, and cancer of the pancreas. Acute pancreatitis occur due to any infection, metabolic disorder or malignant condition often presents with raised levels of pancreatic enzymes like amylase and lipase in the blood. Chronic pancreatitis develops gradually and results in slow destruction of the pancreas, and can lead to other problems like pancreatic insufficiency, bacterial infections, and Type 2 diabetes. The main causes of chronic pancreatitis are gall bladder disease (ductal obstruction) and alcoholism.

Pancreatic Insufficiency

Pancreatic insufficiency is the inability of the pancreas to produce and/or transport enough digestive enzymes to break down food in the intestine and allow its absorption. It typically occurs as a result of progressive pancreatic damage caused by a variety of conditions. Acinal dystrophy and chronic pancreatitis are most common cause of pancreatitis insufficiency in dog. Polyphagia, weight loss, and diarrhea are most common clinical sign observed in affected dog. Vomiting and anorexia are observed in some animals.

Chapter 6

Liver, Kidney and Pancreatic Function Test

Liver Function Test

Liver involve in different kinds of biochemical, synthetic and excretory functions of body. Usually batteries of tests are used to detect and manage liver diseases as no single biochemical test can detect all the functions of liver. These tests are frequently termed "Liver function tests"

Various Uses of Liver Function Tests

- ☆ Screening of liver dysfunction and disorder.
- ☆ To recognize the pattern of liver disease e.g. acute vs. chronic.
- ☆ To assess the severity and predict the outcome of liver diseases.
- ☆ To evaluate therapy or treatment response.

Classification of Liver Function Tests

- ☆ Tests on the basis of metabolism and excretion of biliary pigments.
- ☆ Tests to detect injury to cellular part (serum enzyme tests).
- ☆ Tests to detect the liver's biosynthetic capacity.

Tests on the Basis of Metabolism and Excretion of Biliary Pigments

Bilirubin

- ☆ Bilirubin is an endogenous anion derived mainly from destruction of senescent RBCs (85 per cent) by reticuloendothelial cells in spleen and other haemoproteins (15 per cent, mainly hepatic cytochromes).
- ☆ Porphyrin ring of hemoglobin breaks in to biliverdin, iron and globin.
- ☆ In presence of biliverdin reductase, biliverdin forms bilirubin.

- ☆ This bilirubin is now carried to the plasma where it is loosely bound to albumin and α-1 globulin and this form of bilirubin is termed as free bilirubin.
- ☆ In the liver this bilirubin is conjugate with glucuronic acid in presence of enzyme Glucuronyl transferase. Now it is known as Conjugate bilirubin.
- ☆ Conjugate bilirubin is excreated in to biliary canaliculi by the hepatocye cells and reaches in to small intestine with the help of biliary system.
- ☆ In small intestine bacterial flora converts bilirubin in to urobilinogen (reduced bilirubin).
- ☆ Some part of urobilinogen is excreted through faeces here by oxidized to urobilin which gives orange colour to faeces.
- ☆ Some part of urobilinogen reabsorbed by portal blood system goes to kidney and liver. Kidney removes it as urinary urobilinogen and in liver it is removed by hepatocytes and excreated in to the bile, thus completing the enterohepatic circulation of bile pigment.

Normal Values of Bilirubin in different Species

Species	*Total Bilirubin (mg/dl)*	*Conjugate Bilirubin (mg/dl)*
Cattle	0.01-0.47	0.04-0.44
Dog	0.07-0.61	0.06-0.12
Horse	0.2-2.0	0.0.4
Cat	0.15-0.20	——
Sheep	0-0.39	0-0.27
Goat	0-0.1	——

Van den Bergh's Test

Principle: This test based on chemical reaction which differentiates between conjugated and unconjugated bilirubin in serum. Bilirubin reacts with diazotised sulphanilic acid and produce purple coloured azo bilirubin.

Procedure

1. Take 1 ml of non haemolyzed serum from fasting animal in a graduated centrifuged tube. Add 0.5 ml of diazo reagent (freshly prepared) to side of the tube and overlay on the serum.
2. In direct reaction reddish purple ring is formed in 30 seconds- (Immediate reaction).
3. Shake the tube and add 3 ml of 95 per cent alcohol, and mix.
4. If definite pink color develop, or the color already present from a positive direct test and deepens upon addition of alcohol (positive indirect test).
5. If definite pink color not appear in 15 min and only white turbidity occurs (Negative indirect test)

Interpretations

Total bilirubin: This is measured as the amount, which reacts in 30 minutes after addition of alcohol.

Direct Bilirubin: This is the water-soluble fraction. This is measured by the reaction with diazotized sulfanilic acid in 1 minute and this gives estimation of conjugated bilirubin.

Indirect bilirubin: This fraction is calculated by the difference of the total and direct bilirubin and is a measure of unconjugated fraction of bilirubin.

Laboratory Finding in different Type of Jaundice

Test	*Haemolytic Jaundice*	*Hepatocellular Jaundice*	*Obstructive Jaundice*
Clinical icterus	Present	Present/Absent	Present after 3 days
Colour of stool	Dark	Normal	Clay coloured
Colour of urine	White foam and dark urine	Yellow green foam and dark urine	Dark-yellow-green foam urine
Serum bilirubin			
Indirect reacting	Present	Usually not present	Not Present
Direct reacting	Not present	Usually present	Present
Serum ALP	Normal	Normal, rarely increased	Increased
BSP retention	Normal or less than 50 per cent at 30 min	Increased, greater than 50 per cent at 30 min	Increased
Urine urobilinogen	Increased	Increased	Absent
Coagulation time	Normal	Increased	Increased
Serum albumin	Normal	Decreased	Normal
Serum globulin	Normal	Increased	Normal
Serum transaminase	Normal if no hepatic necrosis	Greatly increased	Early normal, later increased
Blood uric acid	Normal	Increased	Normal
Total serum cholesterol	Normal	Varying	Increased

Hyperbilirubinemia

Hyperbilirubinemia results from a higher-than-normal level of bilirubin in the blood. It results from overproduction/impaired uptake, conjugation or excretion/ regurgitation of unconjugated or conjugated bilirubin from hepatocyte to bile ducts.

Types

Mild Hyperbilirubinemia: Heamolysis or increased breakdown of red blood cells.

Moderate Hyperbilirubinemia: Hepatitis (levels may be moderate or high), long chemotherapy, Biliary stricture (benign or malignant).

High Hyperbilirubinemia: Neonatal hyperbilirubinaemia, large bile duct obstruction, bile duct tumour, severe liver failure.

Tests to Detect Injury to Cellular Part (Serum Enzyme Tests)

Serum Glutamic Pyruvic Transaminase (SGPT)/Alanine Amino-transferase (ALT)

ALT is the enzyme produced within the cells of the liver. The level of ALT abnormality is increased in conditions where cells of the liver have been inflamed or undergone cell death. As the cells are damaged, the ALT leaks into the bloodstream leading to a rise in the serum levels. Any form of hepatic cell damage can result in an elevation in the ALT. ALT is the most sensitive marker for liver cell damage.

$$\text{Alpha-Ketoglutaric Acid + Alanine} \xrightarrow{\text{ALT}} \text{Pyruvic Acid + Glutamic Acid}$$

Increased Level of SGPT Indicates

1. Passive congestion in liver
2. Hepatocellular necrosis
3. Specific diseases like infectious canine hepatitis, leptospirosis, fatty liver changes, liver neoplasia
4. Hepatotoxic drugs- Corticosteroid, Chloramphenicol, Primidone etc.

Serum Glutamic Oxaloacetic Transaminase (SGOT)/Aspartate Aminotransferase (AST)

$$\text{Alpha-ketoglutaric acid + Aspartic Acid} \xrightarrow{\text{AST}} \text{Oxaloacetic Acid+ Glutamic Acid}$$

This enzyme also reflects damage to the hepatic cell. It is less specific for liver disease. It may be elevated and other conditions such as a muscle cells damage and myocardial infarct (heart attack). Although AST is not a specific for liver as the ALT, ratios between ALT and AST are useful to assess the etiology of liver enzyme.

Serum Alkaline Phosphatase (SAP) and Gamma-Glutamyl Transpeptidase (GGT)

Elevation in both alkaline phosphatase and GGT level most often use for interpretation of problem associated with bile duct.

Increases in serum GGT are most often observed with cholestasis and conditions resulting in biliary hyperplasia in all species. Serum GGT activity is an especially useful clinical indicator of cholestasis in horses and cattle because of relatively high liver GGT activity compared to dogs and cats. Serum GGT activity in cats and dogs is often interpreted in conjunction with serum SAP activity. As GGT activity is derived solely from liver whereas serum ALP activity is derived from both bone and liver.

Alkaline phosphatase mainly found in bone (osteoblast), liver and intestinal wall. Higher level is found in young animals with high osteoblastic activity. Liver origin SAP elevation is quite easy to distinguish from bone conditions by elevation of any in liver parenchyma enzyme (AST, ALT, gamma GT) and presence of jaundice.

Sorbitol Dehydrogenase (SDH)

Sorbitol, a polyhydric alcohol derived from glucose. Its conversion into glucose takes place in to glucose in to liver. It is a liver specific enzyme and its level increases in liver necrosis. It is marked of choice in acute liver damage in horses.

Bromsulphthalein (BSP) Dye Test

Bromsulphthalein (BSP) dye test used to detect Hepatocellular damage. After intravenous administration, dye is removed from the circulation by liver and bound to albumin and then excreted in the bile. The rate of reduction in serum concentration of BSP gives a sensitive measure of hepatocellular function.

Clearance Method (Large Animal)

The rate of clearance of dye is determined and reported as half time for the disappearance (T1/2).

Procedure

1. Take 5 ml blood sample from animal before injecting dye.
2. Inject 1 g of BSP solution in animal weighing between 182-545kg.
3. After 5 min, take 2 heparinized blood samples before 12 min preferably at 4 min interval.
4. Separate plasma from blood samples.
5. Add 2 ml each of separated plasma into 3 calorimeter tube.
   - ☆ Tube 1- pre sample plasma.
   - ☆ Tube 2- first post injection sample.
   - ☆ Tube 3- second post injection sample.
6. Now add 1 ml of distilled water and 3 ml of 0.1 N HCl to first tube.
7. Add 3 ml of 0.1N NaOH to each of three tubes and mix it.
8. Read the reading of the tube 2 and 3 against the blank at 565nm in spectrophotometer.
9. Plot the 2 BSP serum concentrations on a semi log paper on the vertical axis with the time in min on horizontal axis.
10. The half time (T $^{1}/_{2}$) is the required for the serum concentration to be halved.

Retention Method (Small Animal)

Retention Method mainly used in small animal for estimating liver function. Calculate the dosage of BSP in mg/dl by weighing the animal body weight in pound. Now body wt divided by 22 gives milliliter of BSP solution to be injected in order to assure the doses of 5 mg/kg body wt.

Procedure

1. Inject slowly the calculated dye intravenously (Cephalic vein).
2. Avoid perivascular infiltration (it causes necrosis of tissue).
3. After 30 min of injection collect 5 ml of blood in heparin in opposite limb vein.
4. Now centrifuge this blood and collect the plasma.
5. Take two cuvettes marked 'test' and 'blank'.
6. Add 1 ml of plasma in each tube.
7. In 'test' tube add 4 ml of 0.1N NaOH and mix it.
8. In 'blank' tube add 4 ml of 0.1 N HCl and mix it.
9. Read the O.D. of 'test' tube at 575 nm setting the zero with blank tube.
10. Refer the O.D. reading to the calibration curve to obtain the dye remaining in the blood after 30 min interval.

Interpretations

Average Clearance Value of BSP in different Animals

Animal	*Time (Average clearance time T (1/2) value*
Dog	Less than 5 per cent retention at 30 min
Horse	2 to 3.7 min
Cattle	2.5 to 4 min
Sheep	2 min

Increased Value

Hepatic disease: Fatty degeneration, Cirrhosis, Toxic injury, Hepatic necrosis and Obstruction in bile duct

Extra hepatic disease: Congestive heart failure, Shock, Fever, Hepatic vein occlusion, Spinal cord injury, Metastasis neoplasm and Amyloidisis

ALT, AST, ALP and BSP Values in different Pathological Conditions of Liver

Conditions	*ALT*	*AST*	*ALP*	*BSP*
Fatty degeneration	+	+	+	+
Passive congestion of liver	N/+	+	+	+
Necrosis	++	+++	++	+++
Biliary obstruction	+	++	+++	+++

N: Normal, +: Increase.

Tests to Detect the Liver's Biosynthetic Capacity

Cholesterol

Cholesterol is steroidal alcohol with lipid like solubility. Cholesterol is found in every cell and forms plasma membranes. It is especially active in liver. Liver esterifies it chiefly with linoleic acid, converts a portion of it in cholic acid and secrete it in the bile.

Normal Range of Cholesterol in different Animals

Animals	*Normal Range (mg/dl)*
Cattle	80-120
Horse	75-140
Dog	125-250
Sheep	50-80
Goat	80-120
Pig	40-60

Interpretations

Hyper Cholesterolemia

1. Intrahepatic or post hepatic cholestasis.
2. In non hepatic cases- Diabetes mellitus, Hyperadrenocorticism, Hypothyroidism, Nephritic syndrome and Pregnancy.

Protein Metabolism

Albumin, globulin and fibrinogen are synthesized from amino acids into liver except gamma globulin which is produced by lymphoreticular system. Total serum protein is usually of little clinical application as albumin value increases then globulin value decreases and total sum of protein will be remaining same. Changes in albumin and globulin value separately give the more reliable interpretation than total.

Albumin: Albumin synthesis is affected not only in liver disease but also by nutritional status, hormonal balance and osmotic pressure. Liver is the only site of synthesis of albumin. Because the half life of albumin in serum is as long as 20 days, the serum albumin level is not a reliable indicator of hepatic protein synthesis in acute liver disease. It level may decreases in chronic liver disease or cirrhosis.

Globulin: Increases in hepatitis and cirrhosis.

Prothombin: Prothrombin synthesis occurs in liver which is key component for blood coagulation cascade. Capillary coagulation time can be used to detect prothrombin deficiencies and liver function. In acute and chronic hepatocellular disease the PT may serve as a prognostic indicator. Deficiency of vitamin K and failure of absorption from intestine due to intestine disease or obstruction in bile duct may also increase clotting time.

Urea and Urea Nitrogen

Urea is produced in liver from the catabolism of protein but it excretion regulate by kidney so urea and urea nitrogen is quite in sensitive as an indicator of liver damage.

Key Marker for various Organs

System	*Marker*	*Organ of Origin*
Hepatocellular	ALT	Liver
	AST	Liver, kidney, muscle, brain, RBC
Cholestatatis	SAP	Bone, liver intestine
	GGT along with SAP	
	Bilirubin	Hepatic or extra hepatic
Liver Mass	Serum albumin	Liver
	Prothrombin Time	Liver

Differential Diagnosis of Cirrhosis and Hepatocellular Damage

Substances	*Cirrhosis*	*Hepatocellular Damage*
Transaminase	Normal/increased	Increased
Bromsulphalein	Increased	Increased
Serum albumin	Decreased	Normal

Kidney Function Test

Kidney function tests is a number of clinical laboratory tests that measure the levels of substances normally regulated by the kidneys can help determine the cause and extent of kidney dysfunction. These tests are done on urine samples, as well as on blood samples.

Purpose of Kidney Function Tests

- ☆ Determine the nature of an impairment of renal function
- ☆ Determine the extent of an impairment of renal function
- ☆ Provide part of evidence upon which a prognosis should be based

Tests that can Aid in Evaluating Kidney Function

1. Blood Urea Nitrogen or Non Protein Nitrogen
2. Creatinine
3. Concentration test
4. Phenolsulpthalein (PSP)
5. Urinanalysis.
   a. Specific gravity
   b. pH

c. Protein
d. Microscopic examination of sediments

Blood Urea Nitrogen

Urea is a by-product of protein metabolism. This waste product is formed in the liver, then filtered from the blood and excreted in the urine by the kidneys. The BUN test measures the amount of nitrogen contained in the urea. High BUN levels can indicate kidney dysfunction, but because blood urea nitrogen is also affected by protein intake and liver function, the test is usually done in conjunction with a blood creatinine, a more specific indicator of kidney function.

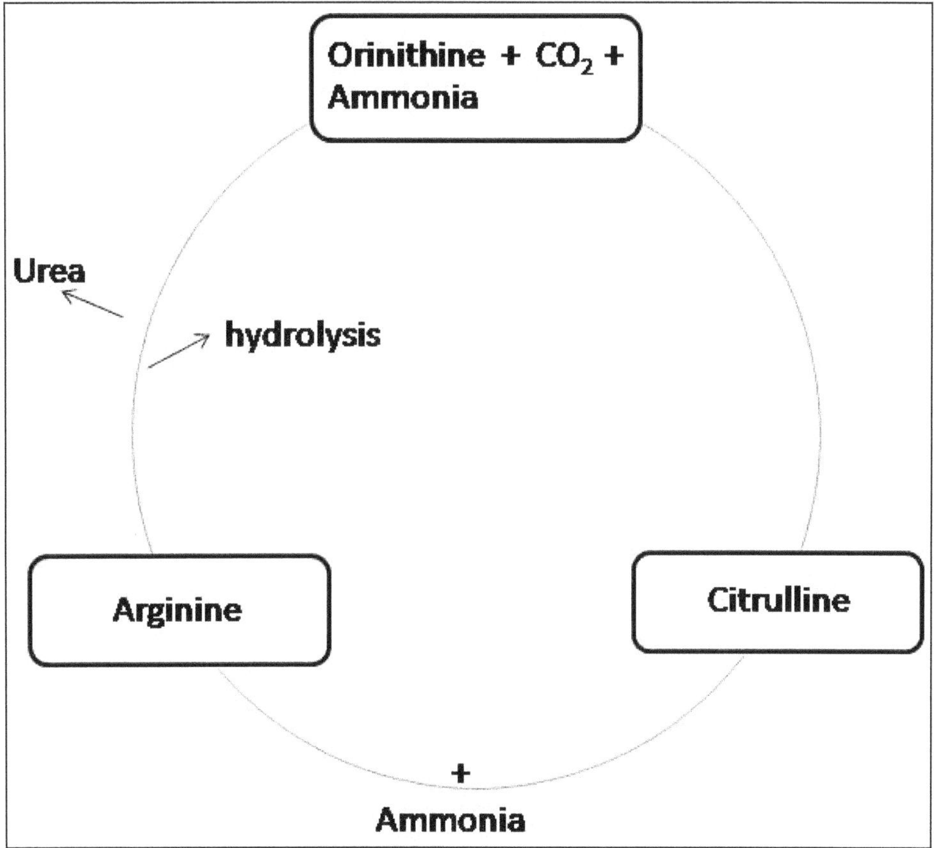

Urea Formation in Liver

Estimations Methods

1. Enzymatic methods
   a. Berthelot Reaction
   b. Neseler's Method
   c. Urease/glutamate dehydrogenose method

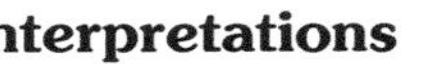

Interpretations

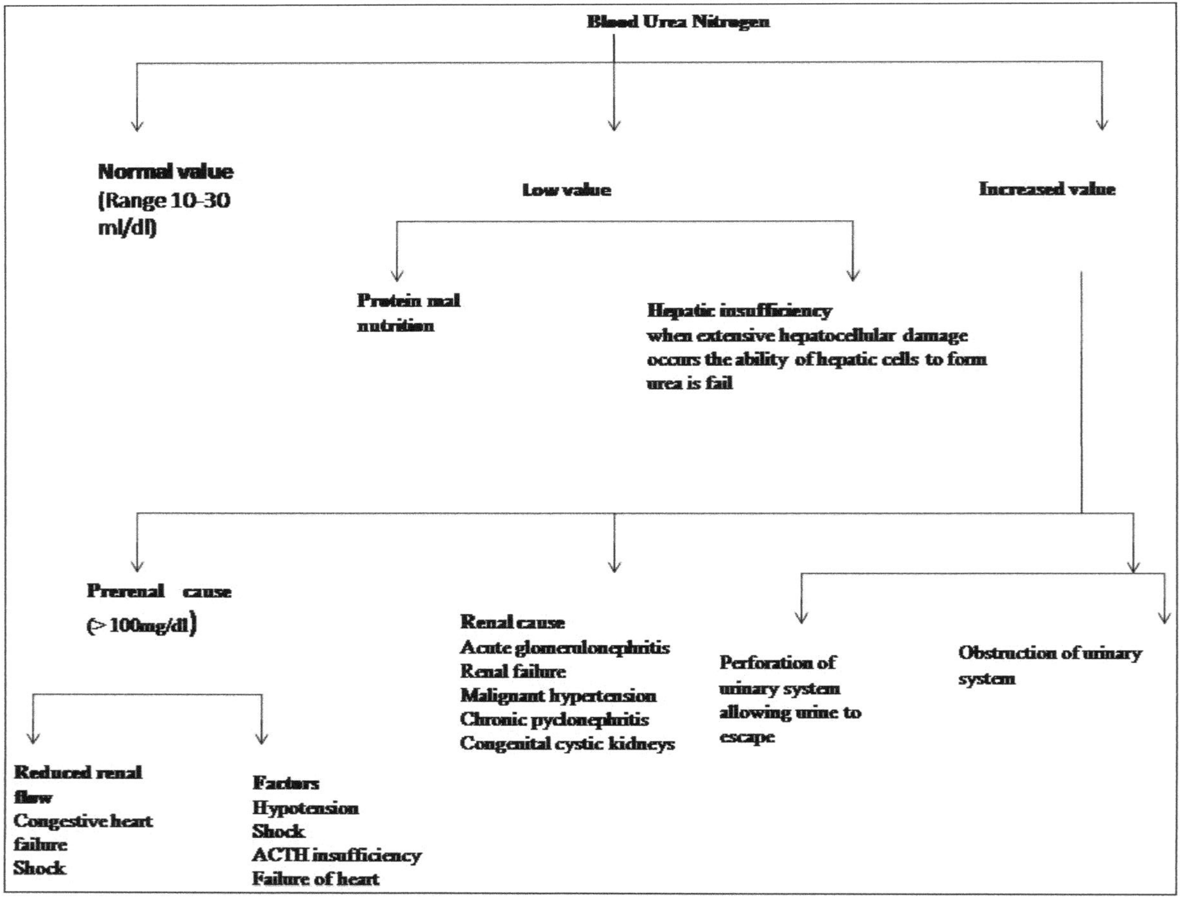
Blood Urea Nitrogen
Normal value
(Range 10-30
ml/dl)
Low value
Increased value
Protein mal
nutrition
Hepatic insufficiency
when extensive hepatocellular damage
occurs the ability of hepatic cells to form
urea is fail
Prerenal cause
(> 100mg/dl)
Renal cause
Acute glomerulonephritis
Renal failure
Malignant hypertension
Chronic pyelonephritis
Congenital cystic kidneys
Perforation of
urinary system
allowing urine to
escape
Obstruction of urinary
system
Reduced renal
flow
Congestive heart
failure
Shock
Factors
Hypotension
Shock
ACTH insufficiency
Failure of heart

2. Kinetic Method: GLDH method
3. Colorimetric Method:Diacetyl Monoxime Method

Creatinine Test

This test measures blood levels of creatinine, a by-product of muscle energy metabolism that, like urea, is filtered from the blood by the kidneys and excreted into the urine. Production of creatinine depends on an individual's muscle mass, which usually fluctuates very little. With normal kidney function, then, the amount of creatinine in the blood remains relatively constant and normal. For this reason, and because creatinine is affected very little by liver function, an elevated blood creatinine is a more sensitive indication of impaired kidney function than the BUN.

ATP + Creatinine → ADP + Phosphocreatine (Muscle Cell)

Normal plasma concentration 150 µmol/l

Method

It is estimated by alkaline picrate method by commercially reagent kits.

Interpretations

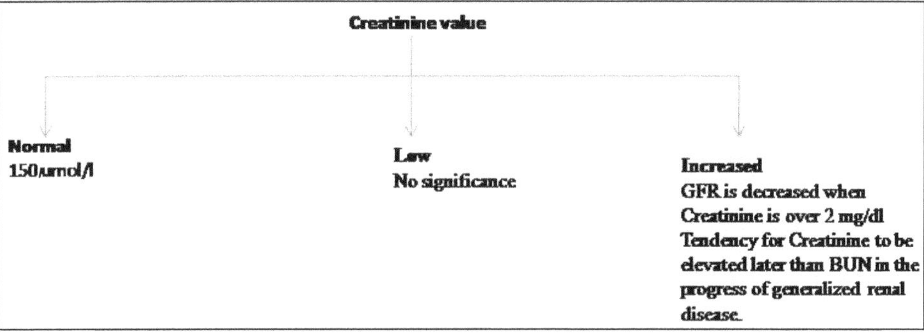

In addition to primary renal disease Creatinine will be elevated in pre-renal and post-renal uremia due to:

1. Impaired blood flow
2. Obstruction in urinary tract

BUN: Creatinine Ratio

Blood urea nitrogen (BUN) and creatinine tests can be used together to find the BUN-to creatinine ratio (BUN: creatinine). High BUN-to-creatinine ratio occurs with sudden (acute) kidney failure and a blockage in the urinary tract (such as a kidney stone). A low BUN-to-creatinine ratio may be caused by a diet low in protein, a severe muscle injury and others.

Pancreatic Function Test

Pancreas is a gland or organ in the digestive and endocrine system of vertebrates. It is both an endocrine (producing several important hormones, including insulin and glucagon), as well as an exocrine gland (secreting pancreatic juice containing digestive enzymes that passes to small intestine.

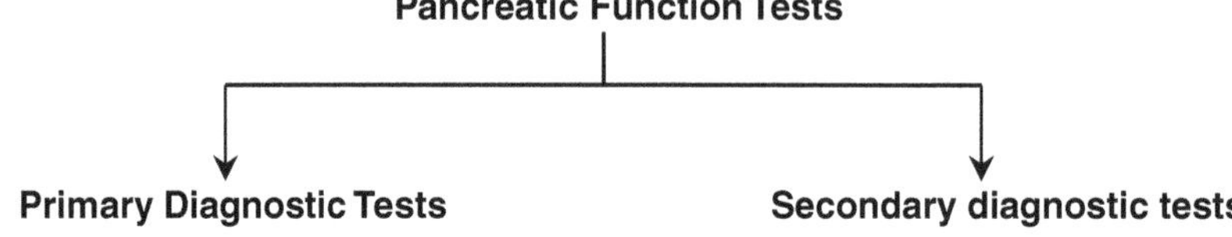

Primary Diagnostic Tests	Secondary diagnostic tests
a. Microscopic examination of faeces of undigested food	a. Serum albumin level
b. Faecal trypsin	b. Serum calcium level
c. Serum lipase determination	c. Prothrombin time
d. Serum amylase determination	d. Blood urea level
e. Blood glucose and glucose tolerance test	e. Serum cholesterol level
f. Absorption test	

Exocrine Pancreatic Dysfunction

This applies almost exclusively in the dog. The condition is not described in herbivores and it is extremely rare in the cat.

Microscopic Examination of Feaces for Undigested Food

It is done for the examination of fat, starch and striated muscle. The existence of steatorrhoea is suggested when the faeces are pale yellow or clay coloured with a foul odour and a glistening appearance. Confirmation of the diagnosis is achieved by adding Sudan III to a homogenous mixture of the faeces and finding red or orange droplets in a smear when examined microscopically. In creatorrhoea the addition of Lugol's solution or tincture of iodine to faeces will delineate the striations in poorly digested muscle fibres.

Feacal Trypsin

Deficiency of pancreatic trypsin is easily revealed by means of a film strip test and gelatin test. Consistently positive results indicate normal trypsin production, whereas the reverse finding suggests pancreatic enzyme deficiency. Trypsin inhibitors and proteolytic enzymes of bacterial origin may give false negative and false positive results respectively.

Film Test (X- Ray Test)

1. Take 9 ml sodium bicarbonate 5 per cent in a test tube
2. Pour feces till 10 ml level in test tube
3. Dip X ray film in this test tube

4. Test tube should be incubated at 37°C for 30 min
5. Now remove the X-ray film and wash under water.

Observations

1. A cleared area on the submerged portion of the film indicates the presence of trypsin.
2. With a deficiency of trypsin the emulsion will only be water marked or partially removed.

Gelatin Test

1. Take 9 ml sodium bicarbonate 5 per cent in a test tube
2. Add fecal up to 10 ml level in test tube
3. Remove 1 ml feces suspension in other test tube
4. Now add 2 ml gelatin (7.5 per cent) in new test tube
5. Add 1 ml sodium bicarbonate (5 per cent)
6. Incubate at 37°C for 1 hour
7. After incubation test tube should be refrigerate for 20 min

Results

1. Failure to gel formation indicates the presence of trypsin, which has digested the gelatin *i.e.* no pancreatic insufficiency
2. Gel formation (coagulation) indicates the absence of trypsin *i.e.* pancreatic insufficiency

Determination of Serum Lipase Level

Elevated Level of Lipase Indicates

- Acute pancreatic necrosis
- Chronic pancreatitis

Determination of Serum Amylase Level

- It is indicative for cases of acute necrotizing pancreatitis
- Slight to moderate non specific increase in serum amylase may be seen o other acute abdominal disorders (including intestinal obstruction)
- Lipase level is more specific than amylase for disease of pancreas.

Endocrine Pancreas Dysfunction

The part of pancreas with endocrine function is made up of a million cell clusters called islets of langerhans. There are following cells

1. **α-cells**: secrete glucagon

2. **β-cells**: secrete insulin
3. **PP cells**: secrete pancreatic polypeptide

Primary Test

1. Serum glucose
2. Urine glucose

Secondary Test

1. Beta hydroxy butyrate: High in ketosis
2. Urine ketones: Positive in ketosis
3. Cholesterol: Invariable elevated in DM
4. ALT and ALP: Elevated when pancreatitis lead to hepatic lipidosis

Blood Glucose Level

Glucose level measured in whole blood, serum or plasma. It is better to collect sample on sodium fluoride.

Tests

Oral glucose tolerance test (detail described in chapter no. 2)

Interpretations

Increase in glucose level indicates acute acute pancreatitis.

Chapter 7

Clinical Enzymology

Fundamental Concept of Enzymology

☆ Alternation in serum enzyme level

It may occur due to:

1. Alteration of the cell membrane permeability due to inflammation, degeneration of the cell, increased cellular activity and fatty metamorphosis.
2. Release of intracellular enzymes into the blood stream after cell necrosis.
3. Impair in clearance of enzyme from the serum.
4. Impair in synthesis by the tissue with resulting decrease in enzyme concentration in the serum.
5. Enzyme production is increased from an extracellular site of activity.

Enzyme Diagnostics

Enzymes are localized in different cellular compartments (cytoplasm, lysosomes, cellular membrane and mitochondrion).

Serum Enzymes are divided into 3 groups

1. **Cellular**
   A. Supernatant or cytoplasm enzymes-
      a. Glutamic pyruvic transaminase
      b. Lactic dehydrogenase
      c. Aldolase
   B. Mitochondrial enzymes-
      a. Glutamic oxaloacetic transaminase- cytoplasm and mitochondria form
      b. Glutamic dehydrogenase

c. Ornithine carbamyl transferase

d. Acid phosphatase

C. Mesosomal enzymes-

a. Cholinesterase

b. Alkaline phosphatase

2. **Secretary:** Enzymes that are synthesized by cells enter the bloodstream and fulfill their specific functions in the circulatory system.
3. **Excretory:** Enzymes that are synthesized by glands of gastro intestinal tract and enter the blood (amylase, lipase).Their determination in blood serum has high clinical significance.

α-Amylase

Pancreas and salivary glands are richest in amylase. High activity of this enzyme also observed in the liver, skeletal muscles, Microvillus of enterocytes, tears, secretion of mammary glands.

Plasma contains two types of α-amylase enzymes

1. Pancreatic (P-type) - Secreted by pancreas (40 per cent)
2. Salivary (S-type) - Secreted by salivary glands (60 per cent)

α- Amylase activity test is very important for diagnosis of pancreatic disease. Two times and more increased activity of α-amylase strongly indicates pancreatic damage.

Indications

- ☆ Acute pancreatitis
- ☆ Haemorrhagic pancreatic necrosis.

Alanine Aminotransferase (ALT)

Also known as glutamic pyruvate transaminase, catalyzes the reversible transamination of L-alanine and 2-oxoglutarate to pyruvate and L-glutamate. ALT predominates in cytoplasm and highest concentration noted in the liver cells. Skeletal muscles, kidneys and heart also contain ALT in lesser amount.

Indications

- ☆ Acute liver and biliary ducts diseases
- ☆ Acute viral hepatitis.

Aspartate Aminotransferase (AST)

Also known as glutamic oxaloacetic transaminase (SGOT) catalyzes the transamination of L-aspartate and 2-oxoglutatarate to oxaloacetate and glutamate. AST are localized both in cytoplasm and in mitochondrion. High concentration of AST is noted in heart and skeletal muscles, liver, kidneys, pancreas and erythrocytes.

Any pathology in these organs leads to significant increase of AST in the blood serum.

Indications

- ☆ Myocardial damage (most significant)
- ☆ Myocardial infarction (along with Creatine Kinase)
- ☆ Acute viral and toxic hepatitis
- ☆ Liver cirrhosis
- ☆ Obstructive jaundice and liver metastasis
- ☆ Progressive muscular dystrophy

AST/ALT Ratio

Its normal value varies between 1–1.3. Ratio decreases in liver diseases and increases in heart diseases. In toxic (alcoholic) liver damage AST activity rises predominantly, where ratio exceeds 2. AST/ALT ratio decreases in viral hepatitis. This ratio increases in obstructive jaundice, cholecystitis, liver cirrhosis, while ALT and AST activity increase slightly.

Alkaline Phosphatase (ALP)

This enzyme is situated on the cellular membrane and takes part in transport of phosphorus. The isoenzymes of alkaline phosphatase (ALP) are produced by intestinal mucous membrane, osteoblasts, biliary ducts, placenta, and mammary gland during lactation. Serum ALP level are most significant for clinical and diagnostic of Bone, liver and placental disease.

For diagnostic purpose classified into 3 types

Bone ALP: Bones ALP is secreted by osteoblasts. Its value increases in serum in bone growth in children, last trimester of pregnancy and reactivation after prolonged immobilization, fractures, deforming ostitis and rickets.

Indications

- ☆ Osteomalacia (malignant bone tumors, multiple myeloma),
- ☆ Tuberculosis of bones,
- ☆ Leukemia.

Liver ALP

There are two isoenzymes.

Indications

First isoenzyme increases in blood serum in biliary obstruction due to decreased elimination of enzyme with bile.

Second isoenzyme increases in hepatocellular pathology (viral hepatitis and liver cirrhosis) (along with ALP).

Intestinal ALP: Originates from enterocytes, enters into the intestinal lumen and partially absorbed in the blood.

Indications: Intestinal diseases accompanied by diarrhoea.

Placental ALP: Most thermostable isoenzyme of ALP. It normally appears in pregnancy but highest activity appears during the third trimester.

Indications: Placental damage in bitches.

Gamma-Glutamyl Transpeptidase (GGT)

GGT is located in cellular membrane, lysosomes, and cytoplasm. Liver and kidney are the main source of serum GGT activity. Small enzyme concentration is detected in Pancreas, intestine, brain, heart, spleen, prostate gland, skeletal muscles In healthy animals serum GGT activity is low. The liver is considered as the main source of normal serum activity, despite the fact that the kidney has the highest level of the enzyme.

This test is much more sensitive than either ALP or the transaminase test in detecting hepatic and hepatobiliary pathology. GGT activity rises on the early stage of the disease and remains high for a long time.

Indications

- ☆ Obstructive Jaundice (most significant)
- ☆ Cholangitis
- ☆ Cholecystitis
- ☆ Parenchymal liver disease (along with ALT)
- ☆ Pancreatic pathology (acute pancreatitis)
- ☆ Renal pathology (pyelonephritis, glomerulonephritis and renal calculi)
- ☆ Alcoholic liver disease in human and its therapy monitoring

Creatine Kinase (CK)

Primarily found in the cytoplasm; however, there is a mitochondrial form that makes up a small percentage of the total CK activity of the cell. Skeletal muscle, brain tissue, prostate, stomach, lungs, urinary bladder, urethra, placenta, thyroid gland are the main sources of serum creatine kinase.

CK is a dimer and consists of 2 protein subunits: Â (brain) and Ì (muscle), which combine to form 3 isoenzymes:

CK-BB (CK-1) – Brain (trace amount)

CK-MB (CK-2) – Cardiac (4–6 per cent)

CK-MM (CK-3) – Muscle (94–96 per cent)

Indications

- ☆ Traumas, Surgical operations
- ☆ Myocardial infarction (most significant), Myocarditis

- ✰ Myopathy, Muscular dystrophy
- ✰ Dermatomyositis, Intoxication, Hypothyroidism
- ✰ Infectious diseases (Typhoid fever)

Lactate Dehydrogenase (LDH)

LDH is present in cytoplasm of every tissue. LDH activity is 500 times higher in the liver, heart, kidneys, skeletal muscles and erythrocytes than serum. Lactate Dehydrogenase (LDH) catalyzes reversible reduction of pyruvate to lactate. LDH consists of two subunits – M (muscle) and Í (heart).

There are 5 isoenzymes in serum, which are distinguished by their subunit composition. They are identified as follows according to decreasing electrophoresis constant.

LDH-1 (H4), – 15–30 per cent: Most specific test for diagnosis of myocardial infarction, teratoma, testicle seminoma, ovarian dysgerminoma.

LDH-2 (H3M1) - 22–50 per cent: Massive platelet destruction (pulmonary embolism, massive.

LDH-3 (H2M2) – 15–30 per cent: Blood transfusions) and lymphatic system involvement, pancreatitis.

LDH-4 (H1M3) - 0–15 per cent: Viral, toxic and traumatic liver damage, exacerbation of chronic hepatitis, in active phase of rheumatism, cardiosclerosis, severe diabetes mellitus, acute nephritis, tumors of the liver, prostate, uterine cervix, mammary gland, intestine.

LDH-5 (M4) –0–15 per cent: Traumas, inflammatory and degenerative muscular diseases and different liver diseases (hepatitis, cirrhosis and others), oncologic diseases (lymphocytic leukemia), active phase of rheumatism, kidney tumors, rejection of kidney transplant, severe diabetes mellitus.

Indications

- ✰ Acute myocardial injury,
- ✰ Haemolysis (erythrocyte damage), hemolytic anaemia or B_{12} - folate deficiency.
- ✰ Injury of kidneys, skeletal muscles, liver, lungs and skin.

Sorbitol Dehydrogenase (SDH)

SDH located in the cytoplasm of cells. The highest concentration of SDH activity is in liver followed by kidney. SDH activity is considered liver specific in all species.

Indications

Dogs: To differentiate traumatic muscle injury from hepatic injury.

Cattle: Hepatic necrosis, hepatic lipidosis, hepatic necrosis, leptospirosis, fascioliasis and hepatic abscessation.

Horses: Hepatic necrosis, lipidosis and cirrhosis.

Glutamate Dehydrogenase (GDH)

GDH is a mitochondrial enzyme and releases in blood only with irreversible cell injury. The liver has by far the highest concentration of GDH activity but lesser amounts are also found in the kidney and small intestine. Determination of GDH activity is best done in conjunction with other hepatic enzymes.

Indication

- ✰ Hepatic necrosis
- ✰ Hepatic lipidosis, and hepatic cirrhosis

Lipase

Lipase is associated with the breakdown of dietary fat and is also present in the pancreas.

Indications

- ✰ Acute pancreatitis and exocrine pancreatic insufficiency in dogs.

Factors Governing the Applications of Enzyme Test

1. Enzyme distribution in the tissue
2. Intracellular localization
3. Release of enzymes from damaged tissue
4. Alterations in enzyme permeability
5. Clearance of enzyme from serum
6. Duration of elevation of enzyme activity in serum
7. Serial serum enzyme patterns
8. Correlation of results with tests other than enzymes

Classifications of Diagnostics Enzyme According to Specificity

Enzymes of High Specificity (Source)	*Enzymes of Moderate Specificity (Source)*	*Enzymes of Low Specificity (Source)*
Glutamic pyruvic trans-aminase: Liver (Small animal)	Glutamic oxaloacetic transa-minase (Liver, heart, skeletal muscle)	Lactic dehydrohydrogenase (all tissue)
Arginine (liver)	Creatinine phosphokinase Skeletal muscle, heart, brain)	Alkaline phosphatase (Liver, bone, intestinal mucosa, placenta, kidney)
Sorbitol dehydrogenase: Liver (horse), kidney	Isocitric dehydrogenase (Liver, heart)	
Aldolase (Muscles)		
Ornithine carbamyl trans-ferase (liver)		
Lipase (Pancreas, intestinal mucosa)		

Chapter 8

Laboratory Evaluation and Diagnosis of Samples for Parasitic Diseases

Purpose of Study

Laboratory diagnosis of any parasitic infection forms an integral part of diagnostic procedures in the evaluation of disease process. Lab examinations of internal parasites should be done routinely which helps in early detection of parasitism and thus preventing infection. Proper examination of faeces provides evidence for an accurate identification of most of the internal parasites.

Limitations of Faecal Examination

- Does not indicate the degree of an infection.
- Absence of eggs and larvae in faeces does not indicate absence of parasites as immature stage of parasite may be presents in intestine.
- Number of eggs/larvae per gram of faeces cannot be correlated with adult nematodes present in animal.

Factors Limit the Accuracy and Significance of a Faecal Egg Count

- Uneven distribution of eggs throughout the faeces.
- The quantity of faeces passed will affect the number of eggs per unit weight.
- Regular fluctuation in faecal egg output.
- Immature worms do not indicate their presence by producing eggs.
- Eggs may not be detected due to low test sensitivity.

- ✰ Host resistance can depress or entirely inhibit the egg production of parasites.
- ✰ Seasonal influence of output of eggs.

Collection of Faecal Samples

- ✰ Collection should be done directly from the rectum of the animal.
- ✰ Middle portion of recently defecated faecal samples should also be taken for sample.
- ✰ In large animals, one should wear gloves and lubricate the hands with water before inserting into rectum.
- ✰ If faeces is not present in rectum, stimulate the mucosa of rectum with finger, the animal will defecate within few minutes.
- ✰ Collect 5-10 g feces in a clear, dry glass or plastic container.
- ✰ For cultural examination, faeces should be collected in sterilized glass vials.
- ✰ In small animals (calves, sheep, goat and dogs) the faeces can be collected by index finger. In poultry, the cloacal swabs are used for examination.

Storage Methods for Preventing the Development and Hatching of Eggs

- ✰ Faeces should be filled up to capacity of container to exclude air from the container.
- ✰ If not possible to examine immediately then faeces should be kept in refrigerator at 4°C. 10 per cent formalin can also be used as preservative.
- ✰ Packing and dispatching of faecal samples should be done in a cool box (ice pack) to avoid the eggs developing and hatching.
- ✰ Do not keep samples in the freezer.

Examination of Faeces

Gross Examination

- ✰ Keep the faecal sample in clean, dry petri dish for gross examination.
- ✰ Spread it properly in the petri dishes with the help of spatula or clean glass rod.
- ✰ Examine colour, consistency, odour and presence of blood, parasite, and segment of parasite or any other foreign material in the faeces.

Microscopic Examination

Routinely the microscopic examination of faeces is performed by following methods:

1. Direct examination.

5. Suspended the sediment in saturated solution of sodium chloride or any of the suspending medium and again centrifuge for 3 minutes at 2000 rpm.
6. Put a drop of fluid from the top on the slide, covered with a cover slip and examined under the microscope.

Reporting the Results

No. Eggs are seen	*Degree of Infection*
Less than 1 egg per microscope field	Occasional
1 to 2 eggs/field	1+
2 to 4 eggs/field	2+
4 to 6 eggs/field	3+
>6 eggs/field	4+

Quantitative Technique of Faecal Examination

Stoll Egg Counting Technique

A method for determining the number of nematode eggs per gram of feces in order to estimate the worm burden in an animal.

45 ml (42 ml water and 3 g feces) x 1/300 = 0.15 ml

Eggs per gram (EPG) = Number of eggs in 0.15 ml X 100 = 1/3 of the total number of eggs in the original 3 grams.

Procedure:

1. Weigh out 3 grams of feaces and put into a dish.
2. Place 42 ml of water in it.
3. Stir the water-feces mixture with the help of spatula.
4. Take 0.15 ml of the suspension and spread over slides.
5. Cover each slide with a long coverslip.
6. Examine the slides for worm eggs.

Calculation

Number of eggs per gram of faeces= Total number of eggs counted 100

McMaster Counting Technique

McMaster counting technique is commonly use for quantitative estimation to determining the number of eggs or oocysts per gram of faeces. This technique can be used to provide a quantitative estimate of egg output for nematodes, cestodes and coccidia.

To separate eggs from faeces a flotation fluid is used in a counting chamber (McMaster) with two compartments.

Requirement

McMaster counting chamber, Beakers or plastic containers, Measuring cylinder, Pasteur pipettes, Balance, a tea strainer or cheesecloth, Stirring device (fork, tongue depressor), (Rubber) teats, Flotation fluid, Microscope.

Procedure

1. Add 4 gram of faeces in a 56 ml of flotation fluid and mixed well.
2. Filter it through a tea strainer into another container.
3. Take some fluid in pasture pipette and placed in McMaster counting chamber to fill the marked area on both side.
4. Leave the counting chamber for 5 minute.
5. Place the counting chamber on microscope at 10X and count the eggs in marked area of both chambers.

Number of eggs per gram (EPG)= (no. of eggs in chamber 1+ no. of eggs in chamber 2) x 50

> The volume of each chamber = 0.15 ml (1 cm X 1 cm X 0.15 cm)
>
> Total volume examined = 0.3 ml.
>
> This is 1/200 of 60 ml (56 ml + 4 g feaces).
>
> For 4 g of faeces, multiplied with 50 which give the final result in eggs per gram of faeces.

Precautions

1. If processing is delayed then eggs can change their appearance to crenated and ghost like.
2. Sugar-salt solution can also change the morphological of eggs.

Faecal Culture

Principle

Many nematodes eggs are similar in morphology so it is very difficult to clearly differentiate it. Diagnosis of specific causative parasite is possible only by culturing the faecal sample and examining the larvae upto the 3rd larvaral stage which has definitive diagnostic morphological feature.

Methods of Faecal Culture

1. Watch Glass Method/Petridish Method
2. Baermann's Method
3. Sporulation of Oocysts of Coccidian

Watch Glass Method/Petridish Method

1. Take a large lump of faeces in watch glass or small petridish.
2. Faeces should not too hard nor too soft. Add sufficient quantity of water or charcoal depending upon consistency.

3. Place this disc in another large petridish having water up to the brim of small petridish.
4. Cover the large petridish with a jar and keep it in the dark at room temperature.
5. Within 7 days larvae can be identified in the water (ova in faeces developed into larvae and migrated in the water).
6. Specific morphology of larvae helps in accurate diagnosis.

Baermann's Method

Principle: The larvae which do not migrate (like lungworm) should be separated by baermann's method. This method is based on active migration of larvae from faeces suspended in water and their collection and identification.

Required equipments: Test tube, Pasteur pipette, Small petridishes, Funnel, Funnel stand, Rubber or Plastic tubing, Rubber band clamp, Cheese cloth, Simple thin stick, Strainer.

Procedure

1. Fit a short piece of tubing which is closed at one end with a clamp to the stem of funnel of appropriate size and support the funnel by a stand.
2. Put a wire gauge in the funnel of the tube and place a double layer cheese cloth over the wire gauge and place 5-10 gram of faecal culture/faeces on it.
3. Distribute the faeces evenly and add water (about 40°C) in the funnel just enough to cover the faecal matter.
4. Allow it to stand for 2 hours during which the larvae actively move out of faeces and ultimately collect by gravitation in the stem of funnel.
5. Remove the water found at the bottom of the stem of the funnel in which will be found all the larvae.

Sporulation of Coccidian Oocysts

1. Keep the faeces containing the coccidial oocyst in a petridish containing 2.5 per cent potassium dichromate solution.
2. Fluid should not exceed than few millimeters.
3. Incubate the faeces at 27°C for a day to a week to allow development of sporocysts and sporozoites.
4. Observe the sporulation of Oocysts each day in the microscope.
5. Identify the various species of coccidian on the basis of sporulation time, micrometry, presence and absence of micropiles.

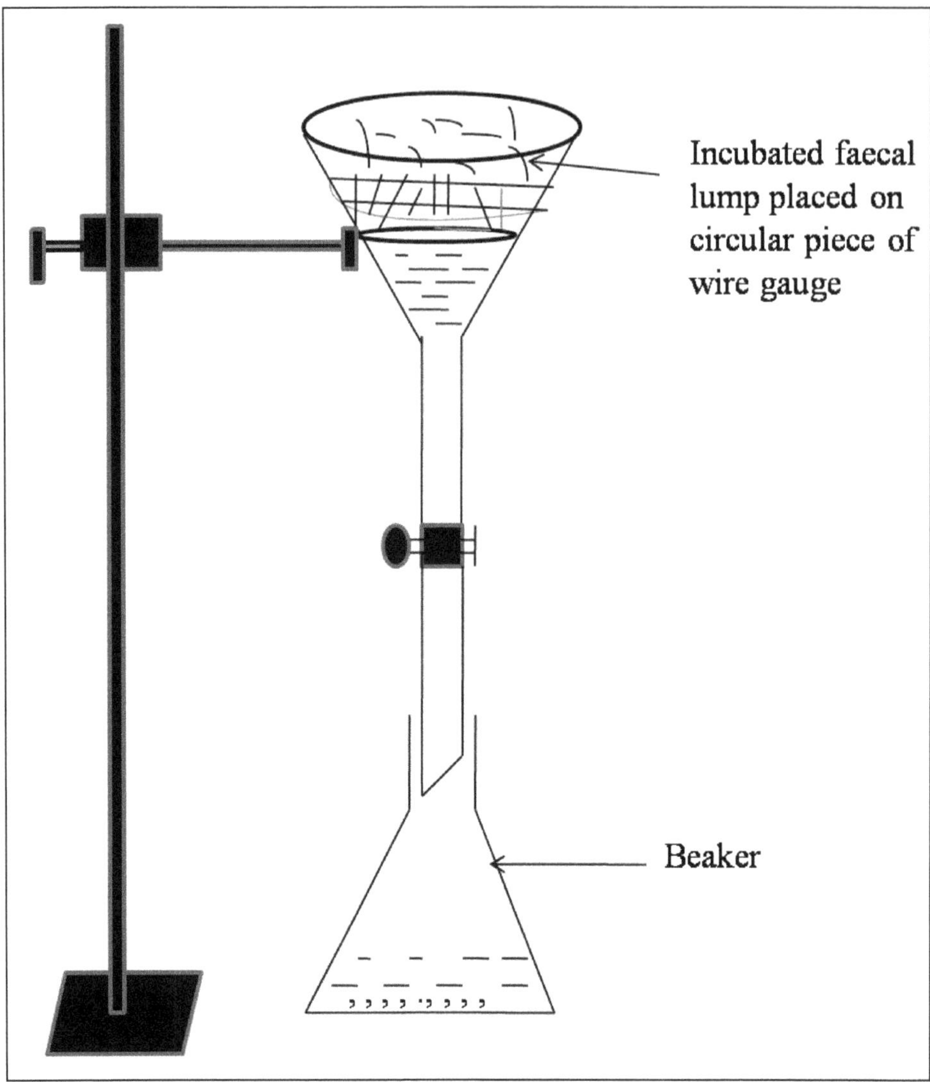

Baermann's Appratus

Diagnosis of Canine Heartworm Infection

Modified Knott method: This is a concentration technique for the laboratory examination of dog blood for microfilariae to increase the sensitivity of direct smear method.

Procedure

1. Add 1 ml freshly-drawn blood to 9 ml 2 per cent formalin (aqueous) in a centrifuge tube.
2. Mix well to lyse red blood cells.

3. Centrifuge for 5 minutes at 1500 rpm.
4. Pour off supernatant fluid by inverting the tube completely.
5. Add a drop of 0.1 per cent aqueous methylene blue.
6. Then stir or mix up the sediment in the bottom of the tube.
7. Mix again and place a drop of the stained mixture on a microscope slide and add a cover slip.
8. Examine under a microscope.

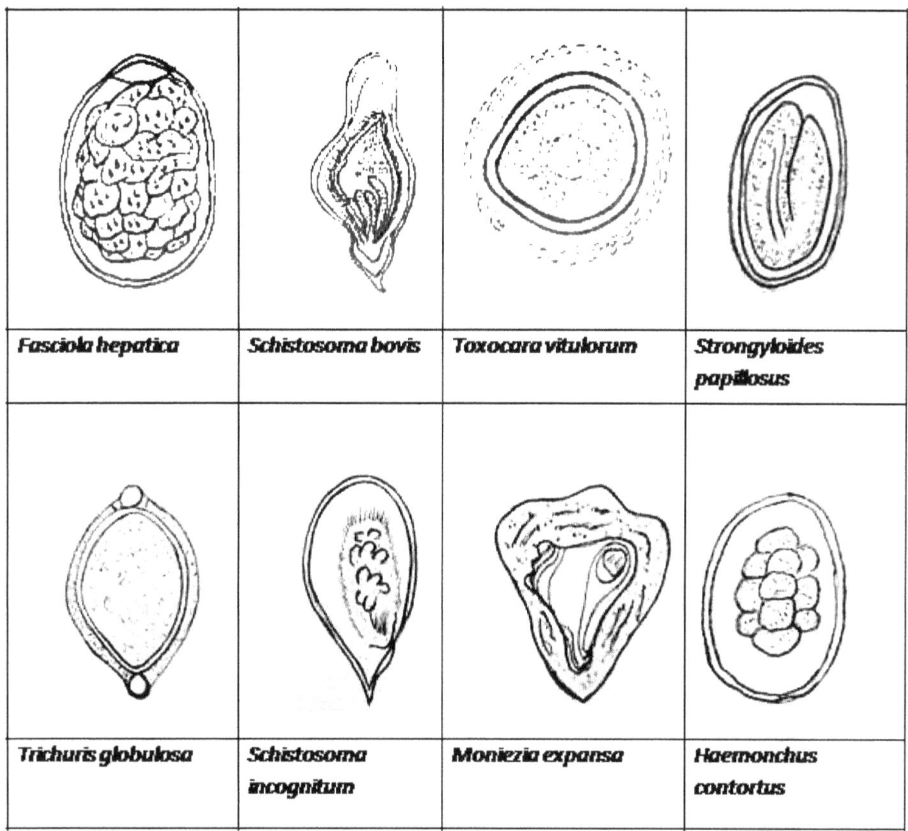

Common parasitic eggs of ruminants

Scratch Diagram of Parasitic Eggs Found in Animals

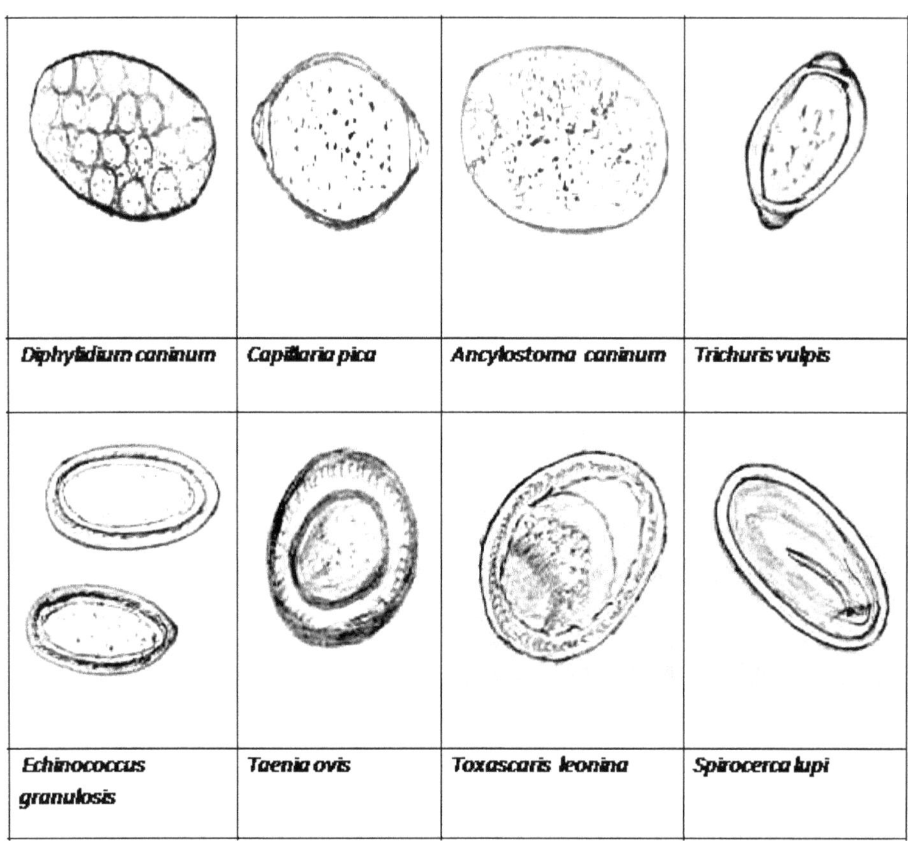

Common parasitic eggs of canines

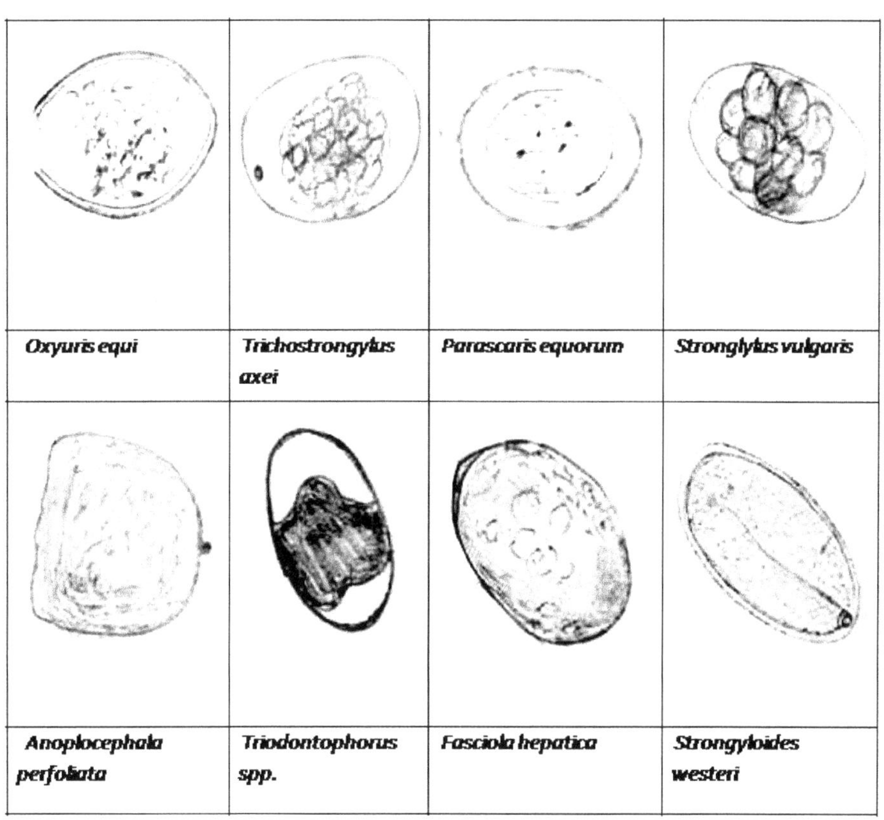

Common parasitic eggs of equines

Chapter 9

Examination of Skin Scraping

The skin scrapping is generally performed in animals for the diagnosis of dermal infections cause by various etiological agents *i.e.* fungal, bacterial, and parasitic. The confirmatory diagnosis of skin disease is made through microscopic examination of skin scraping of animals. Mites and fungus produces skin lesion in most cases.

Collections of Skin Scraping Material in Mange Infestations

1. Identified the affected area (active lesions) and moistened with mineral oil or 10 per cent KOH.
2. Generally the periphery of the lesion contains more parasites than the centre.
3. Press the lesion between the thumb and index finger.
4. Scrap the skin with the edge of a sharp scalpel till bleeding occurs and collect all the debris in to a clean dry container or in container containing 10 per cent NaOH or KOH or glycerin.

Examination Methods for Skin Scraping

1. Direct smear method
2. Sedimentation method
3. Sugar flotation method

Direct Smear Method

1. Place KOH treated skin scraping material on dry and clean glass slide.
2. Add few drop of 10 per cent KOH or NaOH.
3. The scraping are macerated with spatula and covered with cover slip.
4. Examine the slide under low power of microscope.

Sedimentation Method

1. Kept the skin scrapings in 10 per cent KOH or NaOH for 2-4 hours for the digestion of the debris.
2. Gentle heat the test tube till a homogenous suspension formed.
3. Allow it cool.
4. Pour suspension into a centrifuge tube and centrifuge for 10 minutes at 3000 rpm.
5. Pour off the supernatant
6. Examine a drop of the sediment on clean and dry glass slide under the low power of microscope for the presence of mites.

Sugar Flotation Method

1. Keep the skin scrapings in 10 per cent KOH or NaOH for 2-4 hours to digest the debris.
2. Gentle heat the test tube till a homogenous suspension formed and allows cooling.
3. Pour this into a tube and centrifuge for 10 minutes at 3000 rpm.
4. Pour off the supernatant and add distilled water in centrifuge tube to fill it half.
5. Mix the content, now centrifuge tube is filled with saturated sugar solution.
6. Centrifuge the tube at 3000 rpm for 10-15 min.
7. Parasites of mange mites will come over the contents of tube by gravitational force.
8. Take one drop of fluid from the top of the centrifuge tube and placed on clean and dry slide.
9. Place a cover slip and examine under microscope.

Interpretations

Sarcoptes: Globular or round in shape and smaller in size. The legs are shorter and do not project beyond the margins of the body.

Psoroptes: Bigger and elongated in shape. The legs are longer and project beyond the body margins. Coupulatory discs and tubercles are presents at the posterior end of males.

Demodectic: Elongated and worms like appearance. Present in the sebaceous glands and hair follicles.

Skin Scraping from Fungus lesions

1. The fungal examination of skin scraping is indicated when fungal infection is suspected.
2. Swabbed the area with 95 per cent alcohol to remove any saprophytic organism.

3. Take the sample from centre as well as from the periphery of the lesion deeply to include hairs with scalpel moistened with mineral oil.
4. Collect the material in petridishes containing 10 per cent KOH or NaOH.

Methods

Gross Examination

I. Wood's lamp methods

Microscopic Examination

I. Direct examination
II. Periodic acid Schiff (PAS) staining method

Wood's Lamp Method

1. Wood's lamp directed on the intact skin or the scraping collected in petridishes (Wood's lamp has UV light).
2. If fungus of *Microsporum* spp. is present in the lesion, it gives yellow-green fluorescence otherwise no colour will be observed.

Direct Examination

Place the skin scrapings on the glass slide with 1-2 drop of 10 per cent KOH.

Apply Vaseline around the rim of coverslip and put it on the slide

Warm the slide gently over sprit lamp for few seconds.

Examine the slide under microscope for fungus structure (hyphae and spores).

Periodic Acid Schiff (PAS) Staining Method

The skin scrapings are placed on glass slides coated with egg albumin, now slides are gently heated for fixing.

Staining Procedure

1. Keep the slides in 95 per cent alcohol for 1 min.
2. Transfer the slides to 5 per cent periodic acid for 5 min.
3. Place the slides in 0.1 per cent basic fuchsin solution for 2 min.
4. Wash the slides in tap water.
5. Place the slides in zinc sulphate- tartaric acid solution for 10 min.
6. Rinse the slide in tap water.
7. Counter stain with 1 per cent light green for 2 min.
8. Rinse quickly in running tap water.
9. Dehydrate in 90 per cent alcohol and absolute alcohol for 1 min each.
10. Place the slides in absolute alcohol + xylene (1:1) mixture for 1 min.

11. Clear the slides in xylene I and II for 2 min each.
12. Mount in DPX and examine under microscope.

Interpretation

Fungus element will take a bright red or purple red colour.

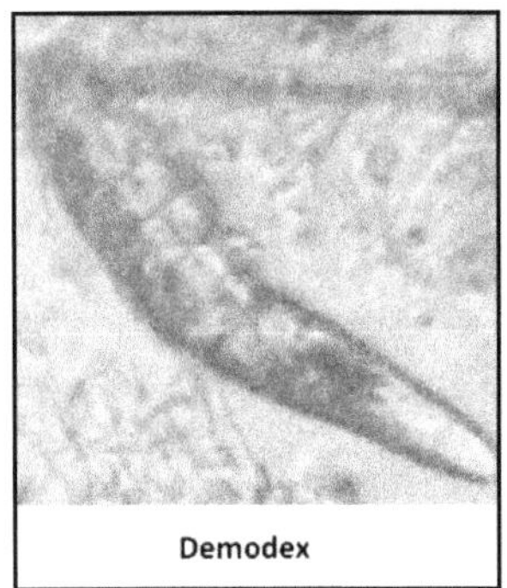

Demodex

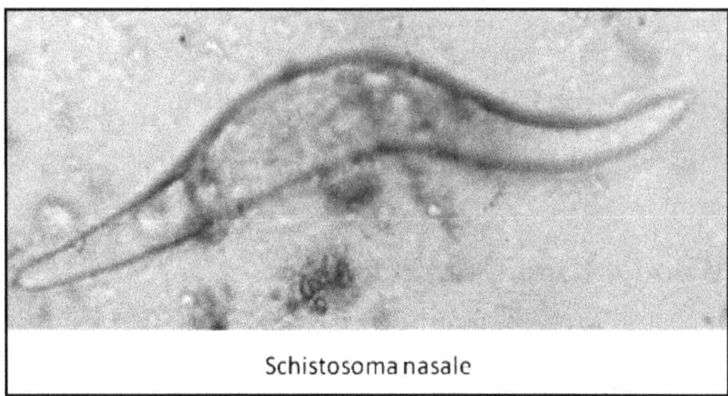

Schistosoma nasale

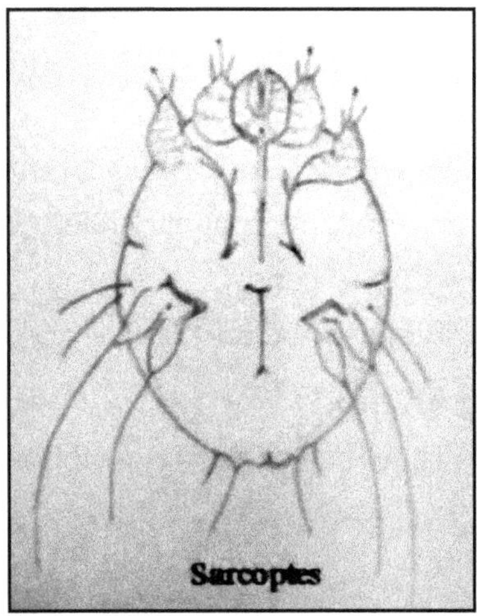

Sarcoptes

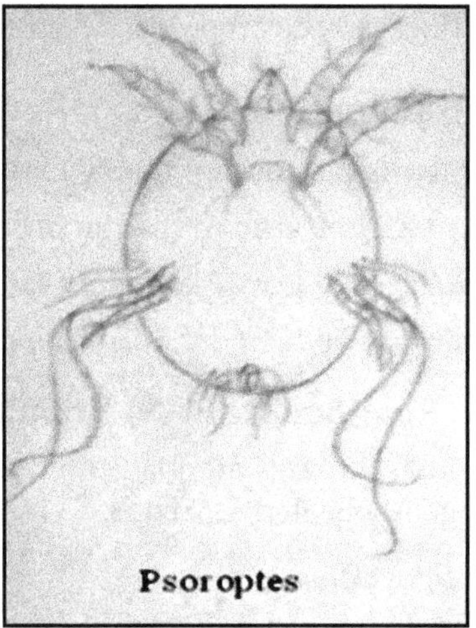

Psoroptes

Chapter 10

Diagnosis of Hemaprotozoan Disease

A number of parasites may be recovered in a blood samples, whole blood, buffy coat preparations or lymph node biopsy material of animals. These include *Trypanosoma* spp., *Babesia* spp., *Thelieria* spp., *Plasmodium* spp., *Microfilaria* spp. and *Leishmania* spp. Blood film examination is the simplest method for detecting trypanosoma and babesia in the affected animals. The thick film provides the greatest sensitivity and should be performed for detecting plasmodium or when less number of circulating parasite present in the blood. Thin films have a lower sensitivity and are primarily used for species identification.

Thick Blood Smear

Thick blood smears are most useful for detecting the presence of parasites, because it examines a larger sample of blood.

Procedure

1. Place a drop of blood on a microscope slide and spread to make an area of 1 -2 cm^2.
2. Air dried the film.

Thin Blood Smear

Procedure

1. Mix the blood sample by rotation
2. Take blood drop on dry grease free slide
3. Make a blood smear with the help of smooth edge spreader.
4. Dry the smear by waving in air and avoids blowing.
5. Fix the smear with methanol for 3 minutes. (not required while using Ramenowsky strain *i.e.* Wright and Leishman)

Characteristic of a Good Blood Smear

- It should be thick at one end thin and feathered at the other.
- The edge of film should be at least 2 mm from the slide edge.
- The smear should have a smooth appearance and should be free from holes.
- Presences of holes indicate grease on slide/spreader.
- There should not be any jerk in it.
- It should cover 2/3 area of slide.
- It shape should be tongue shaped.

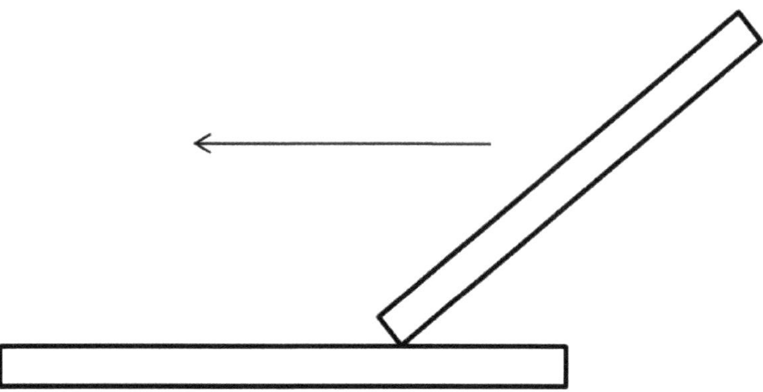

Direct Blood Film (Wet Film)

Wet film examination performs to examine any live parasite present in the blood.

1. Put a one drop of blood on a clean slide.
2. Add a drop of normal saline,
3. Mix it and cover with a cover slip without any air bubble.
4. Examine directly under low power (10X) of a microscope for any live parasite (microfilaria, trypanosomes etc.).

Giemsa Staining Procedure

1. Fix the smear in methanol for 3 minutes.
2. Rinsed the slide in the jar containing diluted Giemsa stain (1: 10) with distilled water/buffered water (pH 6.8).
3. Allow the smear stain for 30 minutes.
4. Drain the excess stain, wash, dry and examine under microscope.

Leishman's Staining Procedure

1. Flood the air dried blood smear with Leishman's stain for 1-3 min.
2. Add double quantity of buffer or distilled water

3. Kept it for 10 min.
4. Wash carefully with tap water, dry it and examine first at low power and then at oil immersion

Wright's Staining Procedure

1. Flood the Wright's stain over the dry smear and allow it for 1 to 3 min.
2. Add equal quantity of buffer (pH 6.6).
3. Mix the stain and buffer by blowing and allow it for 3 to 5 min. Float off the metallic scum with a stream of water. Avoid over washing.
4. Wipe the stain from the under surface of the slide. Air dries the slide and examine under oil emersion.

Precautions

- ✰ Blood sample should be properly mixed by rotation before use.
- ✰ The blood smear should be prepared from fresh blood/anticoagulant added blood preferably EDTA within 15 minutes of blood collection.
- ✰ The smear should be dried by blowing in air.
- ✰ The blood smear should be fixed with methanol if requires transportation/ delay in staining.
- ✰ The Wright's stain should be filtered before use.
- ✰ The container can be used for diluting Giemsa stain as residual stain is desirable.
- ✰ Do not allow stain to dry in Wright's/Giemsa

Interpretations

Trypanosomes- Presence of characteristic organisms with flagellates in the thin or thick blood films.

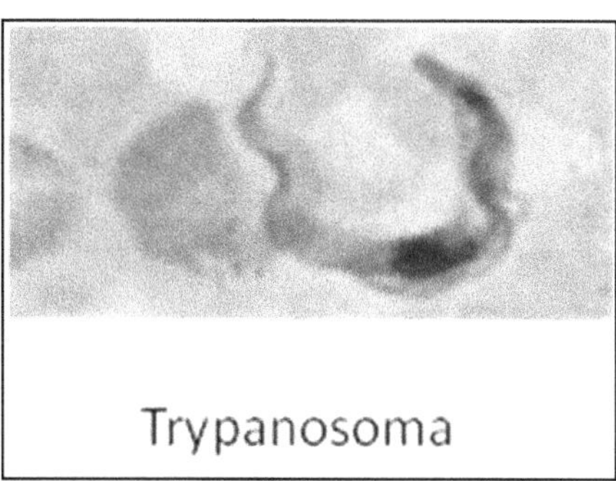

Trypanosoma

Anaplasma- Presence of characteristic organisms in erythrocytes.

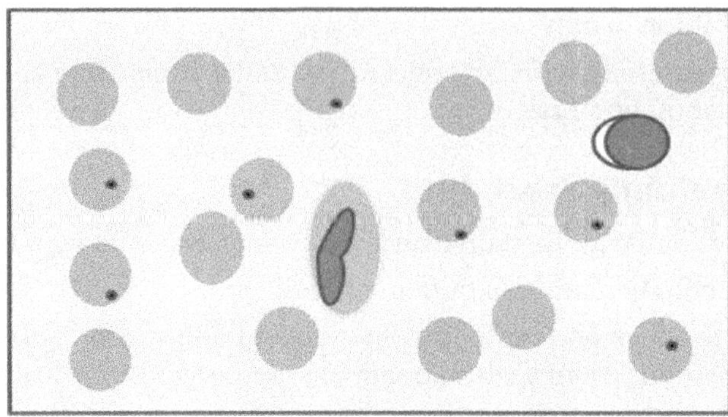

Anaplasma spp.

Babesia- Presence of characteristic piroplasmic stages in the erythrocytes from peripheral blood film.

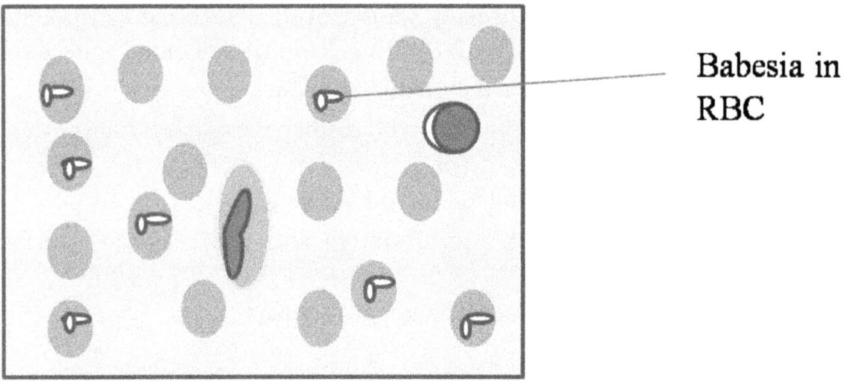

Theileria- Demonstration of Koch's blue bodies in the lymphocytes and monocytes of the lymph node smear or peripheral blood film.

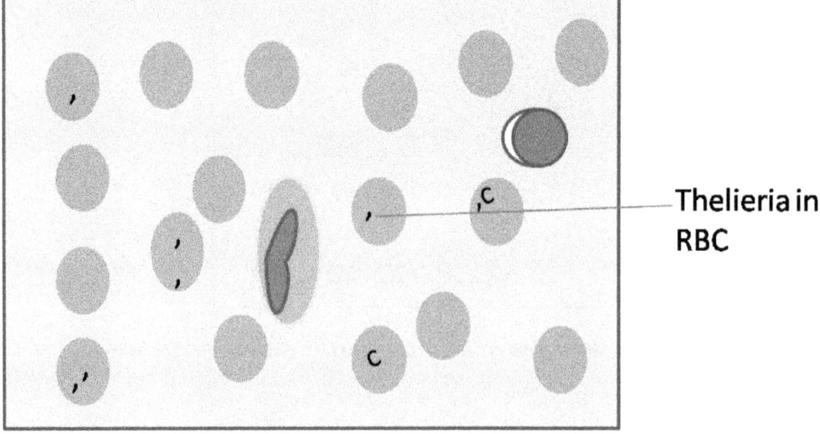

Chapter 11

Haematology

Haematology is the study of the pathophysiology of blood. It uses laboratory procedures to evaluate blood and blood-forming organs. Blood, like any other connective tissue, consists of specialized cells (erythrocytes, leucocytes, and platelets) suspended within a relatively large amount of intracellular fluid (blood plasma). The erythrocytes (red blood cells, RBCs) of humans and other vertebrates contain a respiratory pigment, hemoglobin (Hb), which imparts the characteristic red colour to the cells. In most animals, the mature erythrocytes are flexible biconcave discs that lack nuclei; there are no organelles, ribosomes, or mitochondria. The dogs red blood cells have a typical biconcave shape, whereas in the goat they are more spherical, elliptic in the camel and somewhat sickle-shaped in the deer.

The purpose of blood examination is-

1. To assess the general health of the individual
2. To diagnose the disease
3. To assess the body ability against the infection
4. To evaluate the prognosis of certain disease
5. To give correct treatment
6. To know the efficacy of treatment
7. To know the heredity disease

Haematological Tests for Convenience can be Categorized as

Erythrocyte Related Tests	*Leukocyte Related Tests*	*General/Non-specific*
Haemoglobin estimation	Total leukocyte count	Erythrocyte sedimentation rate
Packed cell volume	Differential leukocyte count	
Total erythrocyte count		

Haemoglobin Estimation

Haemoglobin is a conjugated protein and composed of haeme and globin and makes 95 per cent of its dry weight in the erythrocytes. A primary function of haemoglobin is transport of O_2 from lungs to tissue and CO_2 from tissue to lungs. It also helps in maintaining acid base balance of body by eliminating the CO_2 from lungs. There are four methods of Hb estimation. Two procedures are commonly used for clinical purposes. Both are colorimetric.

1. Direct Method

Haemoglobin is determined by the depth of colour is compared with coloured standard. In this a drop of blood is placed on a filter paper, which is compared with lithographed coloured standard.

i. Tallqvist haemoglobin scale
ii. Dare haemoglobinometer

2. Oxyhaemoglobin Method

3. Cyanmethaemoglobin Method

In alkaline solution ferricyanide converts haemoglobin iron from the ferrous to ferric and form methaemoglobin. Methaemoglobin then combines with potassium cyanide to produce the stable pigment cynamethemoglobin. This is commonly used method to measures almost all types of circulating haemoglobin.

4. Sahli's Acid Haematin Method

Principle: The dilute hydrochloric acid (N/10 HCl) converts the haemoglobin into acid haematin. The resultant brownish yellow colour is matched with the standard comparator or colorimeter.

Requirements

Sahli's haemoglobinometer, it consists of following-

1. Comparator of brownish/amber coloured.
2. Sahli's haemoglobinometer glass tube with marking of gram percent/ percentage of haemoglobin.
3. (N/10) HCl
4. Distilled water
5. Glass stirrer
6. Sahli's pipette having marking of 20 µl

Procedure

1. Mix the anticoagulants added blood in specimen tube by rotation.
2. Place N/10 HCl in the haemoglobin estimated tube up to 10 marks on percentage side, or 2 g percent mark on the other side.
3. Draw the blood exactly up to 20 µl in pipette.

4. Wipe the tip of the pipette with cotton.
5. Introduce the pipette into the tube in which N/10 HCl is taken. Suck the contents in pipette and expel in the HCl several times.
6. The contents should be mixed by circular movements/stirrer and allow to stand for 5- 10 min.
7. Dilute the mixture with distilled water drop by drop, mixing the stirrer till colour matches with the colour the standard.
8. Record the reading in Sahli's tube and record the concentration of Hb as g/100 ml of blood.

Precaution

1. Mix the blood sample by rotation.
2. Wipe out extra blood from external surface of pipette.
3. Allow sufficient time to complete chemical reaction.

Source of Error

1. Using chipped off pipette.
2. Not taking correct quantity of blood.
3. Error in match.
4. Insufficient time as indicated till the development of colour.

Packed Cell Volume (PCV) Estimation/Haematocrit

When a known volume of blood is centrifuged for a constant period of time at a constant period, the percentage of total volume occupied by packed erythrocytes is known as packed cell volume/haematocrit.

Uses

1. Provides a rapid, very useful haemogram of patient.
2. PCV provides rough estimation of total leukocyte count by measuring the thickness of buffy coat.

First **1mm= 10,000** Leukocytes/micro liter, and thereafter each**0.1mm =2000** Leukocytes/micro literThis is an approximate value because there may be error if

1. Marked thrombocytosis occurs.
2. Variability in size of leukocytes cell.
3. PCV as an indicator of the patient's erythrocytes status.

In canine:

1. Total erythrocyte count = PCV/6 (million/cc)

   Haemoglobin = PCV/3 (g/dl)

   These values are approximate value

Methods of Estimation

1. Macrohaematocrit or Wintrobe tube
2. Microhaematocrit method

Macrohaematocrit or Wintrobe Tube Methods

Wintrobe tube- It is a test tube having uniform 3 mm bore and flat bottom. It is calibrated doubly longitudinally with 10 cm scale having millimeter divisions. The scale on the right side is read from bottom to top (0 to 10) for PCV and left in the reverse (10 to 0) for ESR. The tube can hold 1 ml of blood. The percentage volume of each blood compartment is determined by reading directly on the scale. The time and speed of centrifugation are important.

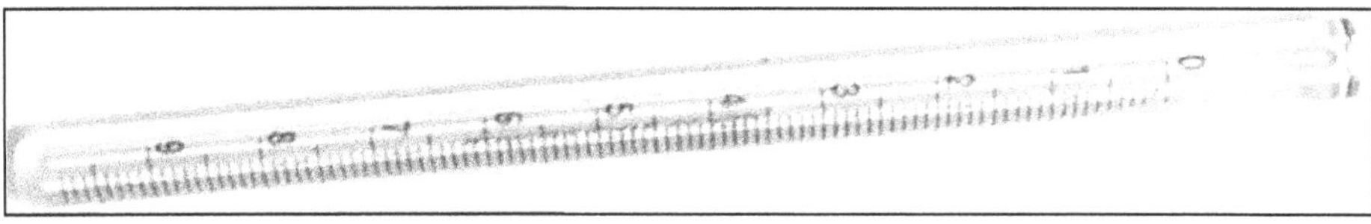

Wintrobe Tube Showing Scaling

Procedure

1. Mix the blood sample thoroughly by circular movements of tube.
2. Take the blood in a syringe with 6" long aspirator needle having blunt end or in a Pasteur pipette.
3. Introduce the needle or Pasteur pipette to the bottom of the tube. Expel the blood slowly and raise the pipette simultaneously as the tube gets filled up to '0' mark exactly.
4. Keep the opening of the needle/Pasteur pipette (Tip) always below the column of blood while filling to avoid air bubble.
5. Place the tube in a centrifuge and rotate at 3000 rpm for 30 min (dog and horses) and 60 min (cattle, sheep, goat and pig).
6. Remove the tube and read the PCV.

Calculations

The erythrocyte will be packed at the bottom and leukocytes and platelets in between (Buffy coat) and the plasma at the top.

$$\text{PCV} = \frac{\text{Height of RBC column in mm}}{\text{Total height of column in mm}} \quad 100 \text{ per cent}$$

Sources of Errors

1. Inadequate centrifugation speeds and time.
2. Not using correct amount of anticoagulant.

Advantages

1. Nature of plasma is appreciated.
2. No costly equipment is needed.
3. Approximately leukocyte count can be estimated.

Disadvantages

1. More amount of blood is required.
2. PCV is not accurate since the more amount of plasma trapped in the RBC.

Microhaematocrit Method

Westergren Tube

Procedure

1. Mix the blood containing anticoagulant by gentle rotation.
2. Apply the one end of capillary tube to the surface of the blood.
3. Due to the capillary action blood rises into the tube. When it is $2/3^{rd}$ full remove the tube and seal the end with the help of plastic or paraffin or with the help of flame.
4. Place the capillary tube into the groove of the special centrifuge in such a way that the sealed end is away from the centre.
5. Fasten the cover of the centrifuge tightly and spin it for 2 min (12000G).
6. The PCV is read with the help of a reader scale supplied along with the instrument.
7. Microcapillary tubes with coated or uncoated oxalates are available in two sizes 7.5 cm X 1.0 mm and 3.2 cm X 0.08 mm
8. Sheep and goats blood require longer centrifugation time (10-12 min). For others animals 5 min time is sufficient.

Advantages

1. Small quantity of blood is required.
2. Shorter time is required for centrifugation.
3. The PCV is more accurate since the amount of trapped plasma between the erythrocytes is negligible.

Disadvantages

1. ESR cannot estimate.
2. Buffy coat is too thin, to be easily interpreted and plasma colour is not appreciable.
3. Specialized and costly centrifuge is needed.

Total Erythrocyte Count Estimation

Haemocytometer Method

Principle: Accurate dilution of a measured quality of blood with a diluting fluid isotonic to blood and count erythrocyte performed in counting chamber.

Requirements

- ☆ Blood samples with anticoagulant.
- ☆ Erythrocyte diluting pipette containing red bead in the bulb. Graded from 0.5-101.

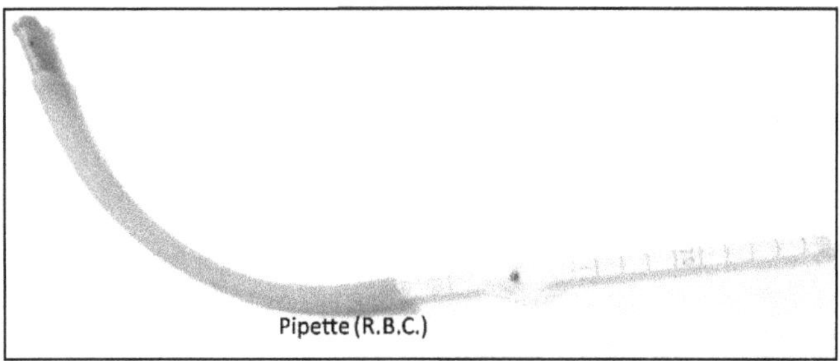
Pipette (R.B.C.)

- ☆ Diluting fluids:
  1. Normal saline
  2. Hayem's solution
  3. Grower's solution
- ☆ Neubauer's chamber

Procedure

1. Mix the blood sample with anticoagulant by rotation.
2. Draw blood in RBC diluting pipette up to 0.5 mark and excess blood be wiped from outside.
3. Draw diluting fluid with steady to the 101 line above the bulb (dilution is 1:200).
4. Mix the contents of pipette for 2-3 min by holding horizontally between the thumb and middle finger.
5. Discard at least 1/3 part of the contents of pipette and wipe off the tip (to remove fluid in capillary portion of the pipette which has not mixed with blood).

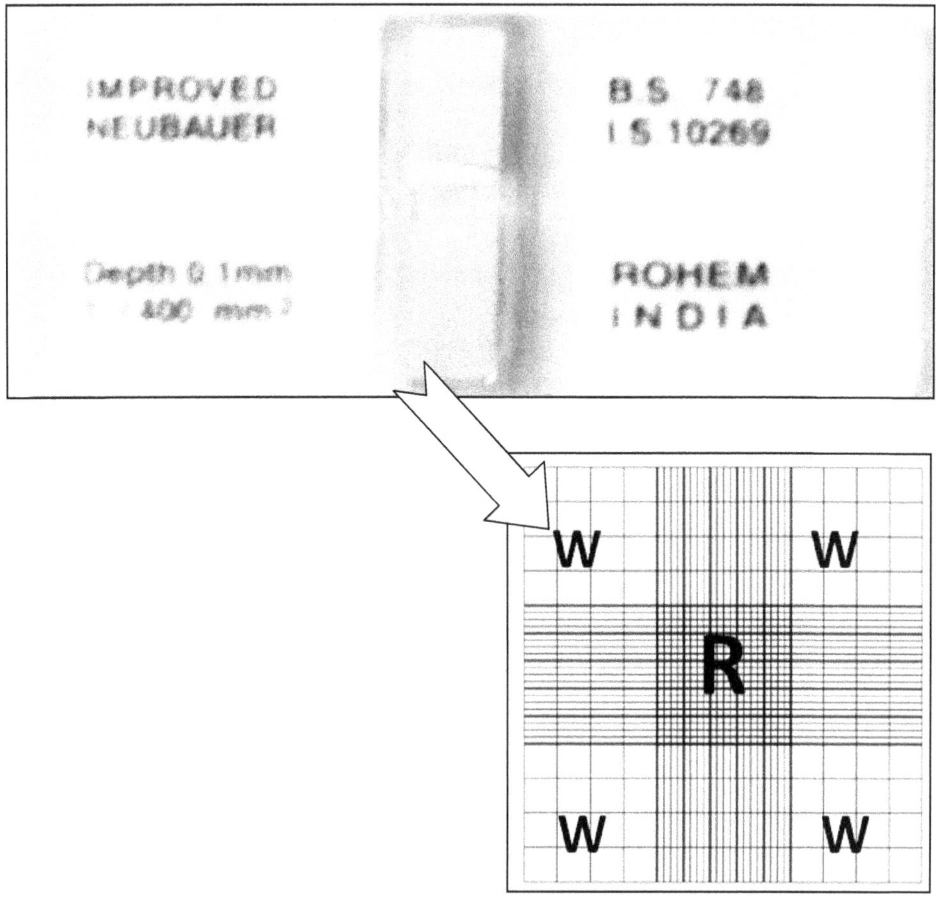

Neubauer's Chamber
(W= counting area for leukocytes; R= counting area for erythrocytes).

6. Load the haemocytometer by touching tip of pipette in space between counting chambers and cover the glass.
7. Allow about 3 min for the cells to set but avoid evaporation.
8. Count cells in Central Square of the 9 large squares. Under high power, count erythrocyte in 5 of the 25 small squares in the central area following principle of double ruling or triple ruling.
9. Variation of more than 10 percent in any of the central 5 squares indicates uneven distribution and requires recharging of haemocytometer.

Calculation

To calculate the number of RBCs in a mm^3 of blood, this formula is used:

RBCs/mm^3 of blood = Total number of RBCs counted in R1-R5 X dilution X 4000

Number of small squares counted

If the blood dilution is 1:200 and if all of the RBCs in the 16 small squares within each of the 5 R squares are counted, the formula is simplified to:

$$\text{RBCs/mm}^3 = \text{Number of RBCs counted x } \frac{200 \times 4000}{5 \times 16}$$

$$= \text{Number of RBCs counted X 10,000}$$

To convert the RBC count per mm3 to SI units (viz. cells per liter), multiply RBC count per mm3 by 10^6 (1liter = 10^6 mm^3).

The mean corpuscular volume (MCV), mean corpuscular hemoglobin concentration (MCHC), and the mean corpuscular hemoglobin (MCH) are three parameters derived from the values for corrected HCt, Hb concentration, and RBC count.

MCHC = hemoglobin (in g/dL) X 100 = grams per deciliter (of RBCs) hematocrit (in per cent)

MCH = hemoglobin (in g/dL) X 10 = grams (per cell) RBC count (in cells/L)

MCH is usually expressed in pg where 1 picogram = 10^{-12} g.

MCV = Hematocrit (as decimal fraction) = # liters

RBC count (in cells/L)

MCV is usually expressed in fl where 1 femtoliter = 10^{-15} L.

Interpretation of Hb, PCV and TEC

Polycythemia- Increased TEC with corresponding increase in Hb and PCV.

Polycythemia may be of two types-

Relative	*Absolute*
Increase number of erythrocytes per unit volume of blood without increase in production.	Increased number of erythrocytes because of increased production of erythrocytes.
Causes:	**Causes:**
1. Dehydration	1. Hypoxia
2. Vomiting	2. High altitude
3. Diarrheas	3. Methaemoglobinemia
4. Excessive sweating	4. Sulphhaemoglobinemia
5. Shift of body fluids to intestinal tissue	5. Chronic lung and heart disease
6. Shock and burns.	6. Increased erythropoietin production, Renal cyst
	7. Hydronephrosis
	8. Cobalt toxicity and local hypoxia.

Oligocythermia (Anaemia)

TEC, Hb and PCV level below than normal.

Acute haemorrhage: Trauma, rupture of blood vessel, coagulation defect.

Distruction of erythrocytes: Bacterial, viral and parasitic infection, autoimmune defect, chemical agents like copper, lead saponin etc., burn, ultraviolet radiation, deficiency of pyruvate kinase and acanthocytosis etc.

Less production of erythrocytes: Disturbance of stem cell proliferation due to panleukopoenia, bone marrow replaced by fat, impaired production of erythropoietin by kidney, and disorder of endocrine glands like thyroid, adrenal, gonads and pituitary.

Disturbance in proliferation and maturation of erythrocyte cells: Deficiency of folic acid and vit B_{12}

Types of Anaemia on the Basis of Cell Size and Amount of Haemoglobin

Microcytic Hypochromic (MCV decreased) - Chronic haemorrhages, Blood sucking parasites, Deficiency of Fe, Cu, Pyridoxine, Riboflavin.

Microcytic Normochromic (MCV decreased) - Bracken fern poisoning, Radiation injury, Poisoning with Soyabean (Trichloroethylene extracted).

Macrocytic Hyperchromatic (MCV increased)- Transitory following acute haemorrhage, Sweet clover poisoning, Bacillary Haemoglobinuria, Leptospirosis, Postparturient Haemoglobinuria, Anaplasmosis, Piroplasmosis, Haemobartnellosis.

Macrocytic Normochromic (MCV increased) - Vit B_{12} deficiency, Folic acid increased bone marrow activity (transitory following acute haemorrhages).

Normocytic Normochromic (MCHC normal) - Anaemia of decreased production, Aplastic anaemia, Inherited enzyme deficiency, acute haemorrhage, Autoimmune disease of new borns, Incompatible blood transfusion.

Normocytic Hypochromic (MCHC decreased) - Stomach worm infection excluding Haemonchus, Leukemia, Hypoplastic anaemias.

Hyperchromic (Normocytic/Macrocytic/Microcytic) - No condition as RBCs can't be supersaturated.

Erythrocytic Sedimentation Rate (ESR) Estimation

ESR is the rate at which red blood cells sediment in a given period of time also known as **Sedimentation Rate; Westergren Sedimentation Rate.** It is measured in millimeter (mm).

Principle

A tube containing blood to which an anticoagulant has been added is place in vertical position; erythrocytes sink because they are heavier than the plasma in which they are suspended. The distance that erythrocytes fall during a given period of time is measured.

Methods

(A) Wintrobe tube method

(B) Westergren method

Wintrobe Tube Method

Requirements

- ☆ Anticoagulant added blood sample.
- ☆ Dry syringe with 4-6 inch long needle (16-18 gauze).
- ☆ Wintrobe tube with steel rack.

Procedure

1. The Wintrobe tube is filled to the 0 mark with long Pasteur pipette on the left side.
2. The tube is placed vertically in appropriate rack.
3. The upper level of sedimentation, erythrocytes is measured in mm on the left scale at time interval for particular animal species as detailed below:

Buffalo/Horse	20 min
Cattle, Sheep and Goat	24 hrs
Dog, cat	1 hrs

4. The results are expressed as fall of R.B.C's in **mm/hr.**

Westergren Method

Requirements

- ☆ Blood sample containing anticoagulant.
- ☆ Westergren tube with stand.

Procedure

1. Fill up the western tube (Total length of 300 mm, 2 mm diameter, a capacity of 1 ml and graduation from 0-200 at 1 mm intervals) up to the 0 mark by aspiration.
2. The tube is fixed in upright position in a special rack with a soft rubber cushion at the bottom so that tube is sealed when inserted.
3. Record the fall of erythrocytes in mm at various intervals as mentioned in Wintrobe tube method.

Rouleaux formation

The RBC's stacked together in long chains like coins.

Causes

Increased serum proteins, particularly fibrinogen and globulins.

Non-specific inflammatory conditions

Increased "acute phase" serum proteins

Sources of Error and Precautions

- ☆ The sample should not be too old (more than two hours) and should not contain excess of anticoagulant.
- ☆ Refrigerated samples should be brought to same temperature since temperature since temperature changes effect ESR and vice-versa.

- ✰ The Wintrobe tube should be perfectly perpendicular.
- ✰ Trapping of air bubbles should be avoided since it affect the rate.
- ✰ The tube should be placed in an area free from any disturbance/vibrations.
- ✰ The tube should be clean and dry.
- ✰ The blood sample should not be haemolysed.

Interpretation

- ✰ It is a non specific test to determine the intensity of disease process in body.
- ✰ Normal ESR does not exclude the possibility of disease.
- ✰ It is more useful in dogs, cat and pigs and not useful in horses and buffalo (very rapid because there is an intense rouleax formation). Rouleax formation (clumping of rages) is seen only to mild degree in cat, pig and dog and not seen in cattle, sheep and goats.

Various Hematological Parameter in different Animal Species

Species	*Haemoglobin Range (Avg)*	*PCV Range (Avg)*	*Total Erythrocyte Count (x $10^6/\mu l$) (Avg)*	*ESR Value (mm/hr)*
Cattle	8-15 (11)	33-48 (37),	5-8(7)	2.25-4
Sheep	9-15 (11.5)	29-38 (34),	8-15 (12)	3-8.5
Goat	8-15 (10)	29-38 (34)	8-17 (13)	2-2.5
Horse	11-19 (14.4)	32-55 (42),	7-13 (9)	61-63
Fowl	8.83-11.3	35-45 (40)	2.18-4.12	1.5
Dog	12-18 (15)	38-53 (45),	7-13 (9)	5-25
Cat	8-15 (12)	24-50 (37),	6-9 (6.8)	15.4

Increased ESR

A. General Conditions

Acute generalized infections, Acute localized infections of serosal membranes peritonitis and pericarditis, Suppurative conditions, malignant neoplasms, Hyperadrenocorticism, Pregnancy (increased fibrinogen), Hypothyroidism, Tissue injury/destruction including surgery.

B. Specific Conditions

Dog: Canine distemper Leptospirosis Pregnancy Pyometra Neoplasms Chronic intestinal nephritis, Infectious canine hepatitis, Endocarditis, Myocarditis Hypothyroidism Trypanosomiasis, Bone fracture.

Horse: Equine infectious anaemia, Stringyloid infection.

Decreased ESR

Dog: Poor nutrition, Excess of immature RBCs and Liver disease

Horse: Hyperglobilinemias

Whole Blood Clotting Time Determination

Capillary Tube Method

Requirements

Capillary tube, filter paper, timer.

Procedure

1. Make a needle puncture in skin of animal
2. Fill the capillary tube with the blood from the puncture site and note the time.
3. Gently break the tube every second until a strand of thread fibrin is seen extending across the gap between the ends of the tube.

Calculation

Coagulation time= Time of appearance of the fibrin stand – Time of first start

Interpretation

Normal Value in different Animals

Cattle	1-5 min
Horse	3-15 min
Sheep	2-6 min
Goat	3-8 min
Canine	3-5 min

Increase Coagulation Time

- ✰ Deficiency of vitamin K deficiency and coagulation factors
- ✰ Thrombocytopenia
- ✰ Bracken fern toxicity

Total Leukocyte Count Determination

The number of leukocytes in peripheral blood in a given unit of blood is total leukocyte count.

Methods

1. **Electronic counting methods-** costly
2. **Placed cell volume methods-** give only approximate count
3. **Haemocytometer methods-** cheap and the best

Haemocytometer Methods

Requirements

- ✰ Anticoagulant added blood sample.
- ✰ Haemocytometer with special cover glass.
- ✰ Pipette (0.5 and 11 mark and white bead in centre)
- ✰ Microscope
- ✰ Diluting fluid
  - § (N/10) HCl
  - § Turk's Fluids

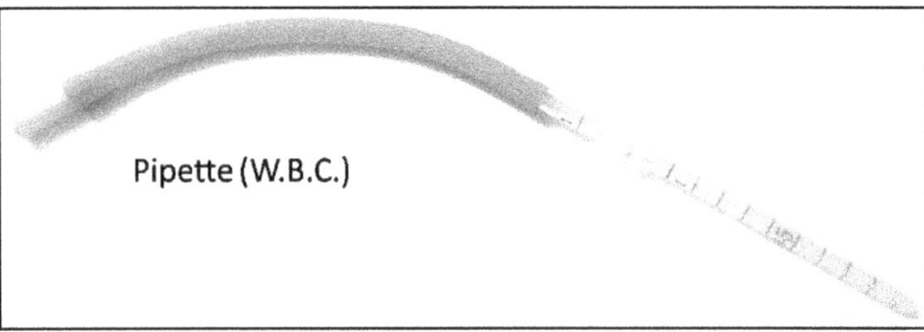

Procedure

1. Mix the blood sample by rotation.
2. Take the blood in WBC diluting pipette (after attaching with rubber tubing) up to 0.5 mark and wipe blood from the outside.
3. Draw diluting fluid steadily to the 11 mark above the blood.
4. Mix the content the pipette keeping it horizontal for 2-3 minutes.
5. Discard first 2-3 drops (1/3 parts) from the pipette before filling the counting chamber.
6. Load the haemocytometer by touching the tip of pipette in space between edge and cover glass.
7. Allow leukocytes to settle for 2 minutes and also for lysis of erythrocytes.
8. Count the cells under low power magnification (10X) in four corner large squares (each is divided in 16 small squares) by following the exclusion principle of cells counting along the line as discussed in TEC.

Calculation

Area of one smallest square = 1/4 1/4 = 1/16mm^2

Depth of the counting chamber = 1/10mm

Volume of one smallest square = 1/10mm 1/16mm^2 = 1/160mm^3

4 corners 16 SS = 64 SS 1/160mm^3 = 64/160mm^3 = 0.4mm^3

Total volume = 64 SS 1/160mm^3 = 64/160mm^3 = 0.4mm^3

Dilution = 1:20

Therefore, Total WBC = cell counted/dilution volume

= cell counted/1:20 0.4

= cell counted 20/0.4

= cell counted 50

Differential Leukocyte Count (DLC) Determination

The differential count can be made by counting 100 cells in well stained blood smear and classifying different cells the examination of well stained blood smear by a knowledgeable observer can provide more valuable information than any other single laboratory test. There are two methods for DLC examination:

1. **Slide method**
2. **Coverslip method**

> In poultry heterophiles is present in place of neutrophiles
>
> ✰ Have lance-shaped granules,
>
> ✰ Lack myeloperoxidase and alkaline phosphatase,
>
> ✰ Very phagocytic.

Requirements

- ✰ Blood sample collected in anticoagulant preferably with EDTA/Fresh blood
- ✰ Dry and clean slide
- ✰ Strains- Giemsa, Wrights, Leishman.
- ✰ Methanol/ethyl alcohol/formaldehyde.
- ✰ Applicator stick/capillary tube.
- ✰ Cell counter.

Procedure

1. Mix the blood sample by rotation.
2. Take blood on dry grease free smooth edged slide near blood drop to $2/3^{rd}$ of slide, the spreader is gently pushed to draw blood smear.
3. The smear is dried by waving in air and avoids blowing.
4. Fix the smear with methanol (not required while using Ramenowsky strain *i.e.* Wright and Leishman) for 3 minutes.

Giemsa Staining

1. Fix the smear in methanol for 3 minutes if not already fixed and dry.
2. Flood the slide placed over glass bars/use Couplin jar for using diluted Giemsa stain (1: 10) with distilled water/buffered water (pH 6.8).
3. Allow the smear for stain for 30 minutes. For rapid staining of 10-15 minutes Giemsa can be used in dilution.
4. Drain the excess stain, wash, dry and examine.

Leishman's Stain

1. Cover the blood smear with Leishman's stain for 1-3 min.
2. Add double quantity of buffer of pH 6.6 and mix by blowing air. When properly mixed a greenish metallic sheen will form. The buffer makes the stain to penetrate into cells.
3. Kept it for 10 min.
4. Replace with distilled water.
5. Differentiate in distilled water for 1min.
6. Wipe the bottom of slide and dry at once.

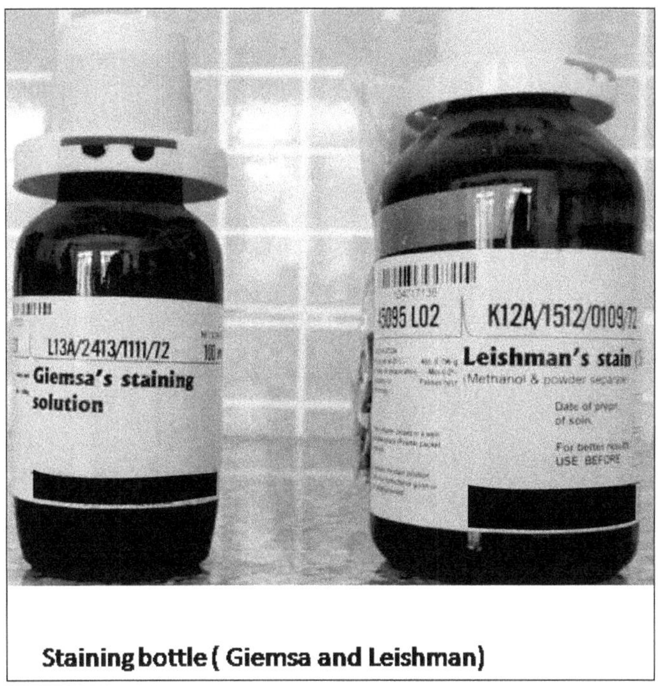

Staining bottle (Giemsa and Leishman)

Wright's Stain

1. Cover the dry smear with Wright's stain and allow it for 1 to 3 min.
2. Add equal quantity of buffer of pH 6.6.
3. Mix the blowing and allow it for 3 to 5 min. Float off the metallic scum with a stream of water. Do not pour off the stain before washing lest a precipitate may from on the slide. Avoid over washing.
4. Wipe the stain from the under surface of the slide while wet. Dry it and examine under oil emersion.

Interpretation of TLC and DLC

Increase in total leukocytes count: Cancer of bone marrow, excitement and muscular activity.

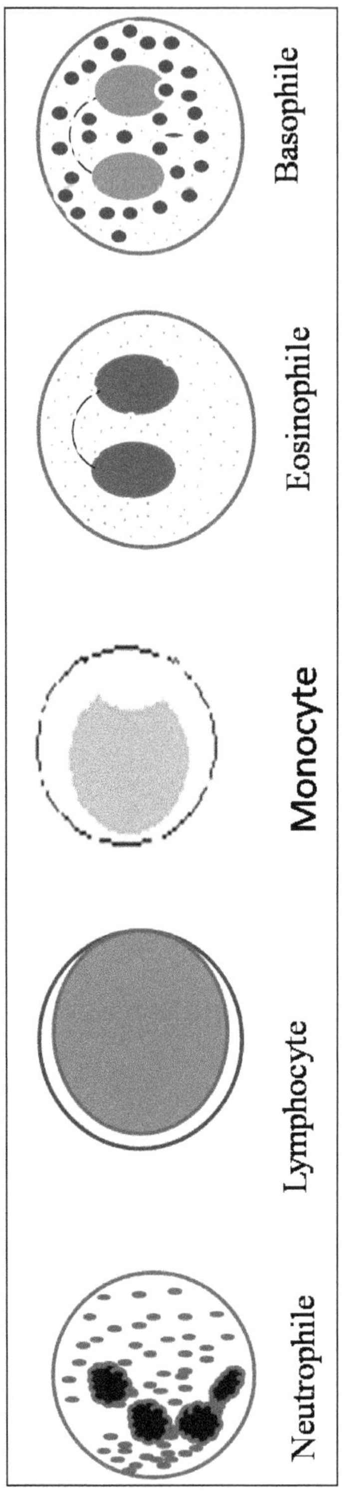
Neutrophile
Lymphocyte
Monocyte
Eosinophile
Basophile

Leucopenia (low leukocyte count): Viral diseases (canine distemper, infectious canine hepatitis), early bacterial infection, parasitic infection (Toxoplasmosis), abnormality in bone marrow.

Neutropenia (low neutrophils count): Bacterial/viral infections, bone marrow depression, deficiency of folic acid and Vit $B_{12,}$ shock etc.

Eosinopenia (Decreased in absolute count of eosinophils): Trauma, stress, intoxication and hyperadrenocorticism.

Lymphopenia (Decrease in absolute count of lymphocytes): Viral diseases (like Canine distemper, Bovine viral diarrhea), hyper adrenocorticism, radiation, immune suppressive drugs, chronic enteric disease.

Leukocytosis (Increase in absolute count of leukocytes): Localized/generalized infections aute blood loss, haemorrhage, strenuous exercise, convulsion, excitement, fear, digestion and pregnancy, uremia, acidosis, diabetes, chemicals (Pb, Hg) foreign protein reaction and snake/insect venom, Infraction, burn, gangrene, neoplasm, adrenal corticoids, trauma particularly following surgery.

Neutrophilia (Increase in absolute count of neurophiles): Inflammation, Bacterial, rickettsial, mycotic and parasitic infection, non inflammatory neutrophilia with systemic stress associated with endogenous release of corticosteroid (trauma, neoplasia, intoxication, surgical procedures, Hyperadrenocorticism, metabolic and endocrine disorders).

Shift to left: Increase in immature neutrophils (above 6 per cent of TLC) poor prognosis.

Shift to right: Increase in number of mature neutrophils (Horse shoe or multiplied nucleus).

Schilling index use to express the increase in mature/immature neutrophils.

Lymphocytosis(Increase in absolute count of lymphocytes): Chronic infections, after vaccination, autoimmune disease, physiological in calves and kittens, lymphadenitis/lymphangitishypoadrenocortism, relative lymphocytes along with leucopenia and neutropenia.

Eosinophilia (Increase in absolute count of eosinophils): Allergic (skin allergies, Allergic bronchitis, anaphylactic reaction), Parasitism (Hookworm, lungworm, Trichinosis, Fascioliasis, Strongylosis), Adrenocortical insufficiency, Diseases of mast cells rich organ (skin, lung GIT and female genital tract during estrus), Eosinophilic myositis, Protozoa: (Babesiosis, theileriasis) Chronic condition of skin (subcutaneous), lung, GIT uterus scrotum and serosal lining.

Monocytosis (Increase in absolute count of monocytes): All chronic supportive diseases, Corticoids in dogs and cattle, Recovery/late phase of acute disease, Granulomatous conditions- Tuberculosis, Brucellosis, Mycotic (Systemic) infections, Disease with tissue debris: hemorrhages exudates in cavities, Pyometra, retained placenta Monocytic leukemia in canine and stress.

Basophilia (Increase in absolute count of basophils): Associated with Eosinophilia *e.g.* heart worms, chronic respiratory disease, Basophilic leukemia, Hypothyroidism, Hyperadrenocorticism in dogs.

Normal Haemogram of Domestic Animals, Poultry and Man

Species	*TLC ($x10^3$)*	*Neutrophile (per cent)*	*Lymphocyte (per cent)*	*Monocyte (per cent)*	*Eosinophiles (per cent)*	*Basophiles (per cent)*
Buffalo	10.61	43-45	45-48	–	3-4	–
Cattle	4-12 (5.6)	15-45	48-75	2-7	2-15	0-2
Sheep	4-12 (5.6)	10-50	40-75	1-5	1-8	0-3
Goat	6-16 (12)	30-48	50-70	1-4	3-8	0-2
Pig	11-22(16)	28-47	39-60	2-10	1-11	0-2
Horse	7-14(8.8)	30-65	25-70	1-8	1-10	0-3
Dog	5.6-19(19.7)	60-75	12-30	3-9	2-10	rare
Cat	8-25(13.8)	35-75	22-55	1-4	2-10	rare
Fowl	20-35(33.3)	29.5-37.3	48.9-58.4	9.7-10.2	1.7	0.7-2
Man	5-10	55-70	25-70	3-7	1-4	0.1

Proforma for Filling of Hematological Report of Animals.

Blood Examination Report

Date .... case no. ....

Name and address of the owner:

....

....

Species: .... Breed: .... Sex: .... Age: ....

History/ symptom/ treatment, if any:

....

....

....

Hematology	Blood chemistry
Total erythrocyte count:	Blood Glucose:.........................mg%
....million/ Cu mm	
Total leukocyte count:	Total serum cholesterol: ....mg%
..................................Thousand/ Cu mm	Total serum protein: .... mg%
haemoglobin: ....(gm%)	Serum albumin: .... mg%
	Blood urea nitrogen: ....mg%
	Serum Creatinine: ....mg%
ESR: .... (mm/hr)	Serum uric acid: ....mg%
Haematocrit:	SGOT: ....units/ml
Differential leukocyte count (%):	SGPT: ....units/ ml
Neutrophils:	Alkaline Phosphatase: ....units/ ml
....	
Lymphocytes:	Serum bilirubin: .... mg%
....	
Basophiles:	
Eosinophiles:	
	Pathologist

Chapter 12

Preparation of Microscopic Slides from Tissues Collected for Diagnosis and its Histopathological Interpretation

Histopathology

Histopathology is the branch of pathology which concerns with the pathological alternations in tissue as a result of disease. It is mostly effective technique in diagnosis of cancer. Most of histopathological techniques simulate with the normal histological structure. Tissue must be processed in the manner that it will provide maximum information for the demonstration of minute histological changes. This technique is useful for clinicians in diagnosis of diseases.

Scope of Histopathology

1. Useful in establish the pathogenesis and pathology of any diseases.
2. Best alternate to diagnose the disease of very long incubation period, low immune response and fastidious organism.
3. Histopathological slide can be stored for long time.

Steps in Histopathological Techniques of Sectioning

1. Collection of tissue
2. Fixation
3. Washing
4. Dehydration
5. Clearing
6. Impregnation
7. Casting of blocks

8. Trimming
9. Section cutting
10. Staining

Collection of Tissue

It should be kept in mind that the representative sample will give the reliable diagnosis. Following points must be kept in mind at the time of tissue collection-

- Sample should be collected as soon as possible in dead animal because it will not give a true picture of microscopic lesion when autolytic changes start in dead body.
- Representative tissue piece should have the part of lesion and a part of normal tissue.
- Do not destroy the normal architecture of tissue during tissue cutting.
- After collection keep the tissue immediately into the fixative.
- For homogenous and smooth fixation size of tissue should not be more than 5 mm.
- Covering of organs like liver, kidney and brain etc provide useful information on histopathological examination so these organs should be collected with their covering (brain with meninges, liver and kidney with their capsule).

> Whole mounts- These are preparation of entire animal eg. fungus, parasite.
>
> **Sections-** The majority of the preparations in histology are sections. The tissue is cut in about 3-5 mm thick pieces processed and 5 microns thick sections are cut on a microtome.

Fixation

- After collection of sample, fixation of tissue is necessary to prevent autolysis and purification by saprophytes.
- Tissue should be kept in fixative for 24-48 hours at room temperature.
- Tissue fixation is also necessary to prevents architecture damage of tissue and shrinkage.
- The volume of the fixative added is 10 times the volume of the tissues.
- The choice of fixative depends on the type of investigation required.

> **Fixation of tissue prevents**
>
> **Autolysis** (lysis or dissolution of cells by enzymatic action probably as a result of rupture of lysosomes).
>
> **Putrefaction** (The breakdown of tissue by bacterial action often with formation of gas).

Routine Fixatives

- Formal saline (10 per cent formaldehyde in 0.85 per cent sodium chloride solution).

- ☆ Buffered formalin (is better than formal saline because of its tolerance capacity, tissue can be left for longer periods without excessive hardening and damage).

Special Fixatives

- ☆ Zenker's fluid- Nucleus and connective tissue stain sharply.
- ☆ Bouin's fluid- Nucleus stains excellently because of rapid penetration and it is useful for nervous tissue.

Washing

- ☆ After fixation tissue should be kept in running tap water overnight (12 hours) to remove the formalin from tissue by placing it in a small capsule or gauze.

Dehydration

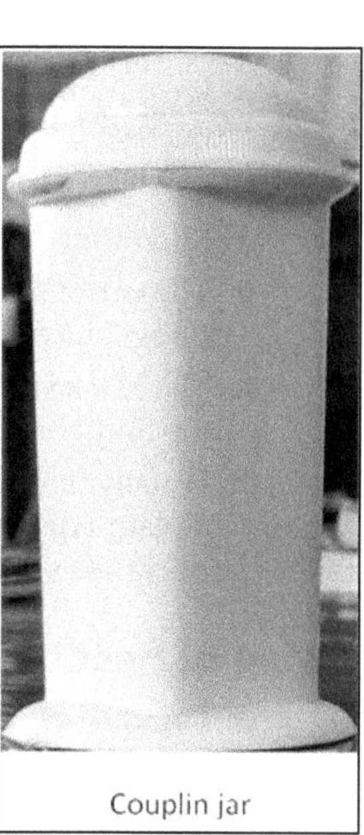

Couplin jar

- ☆ Dehydration is done in ascending series of graded ethanol of 50 per cent, 70 per cent, 80 per cent, 90 per cent, 95 per cent, absolute ethanol I and absolute ethanol II for one hour each in Couplin jar.
- ☆ To increase the process of dehydration the tissue block should be agitated mechanically or in automatic tissue processor.
- ☆ Volume of alcohol should be at least 50 times more than tissue placed for dehydration process.

Cleaning

- ☆ Xylene is being used for clearing of tissue block.
- ☆ After dehydration first clearing is done in mixture of ethanol and xylene in 1:1 ratio, followed by xylene I and xylene II for one hour each.

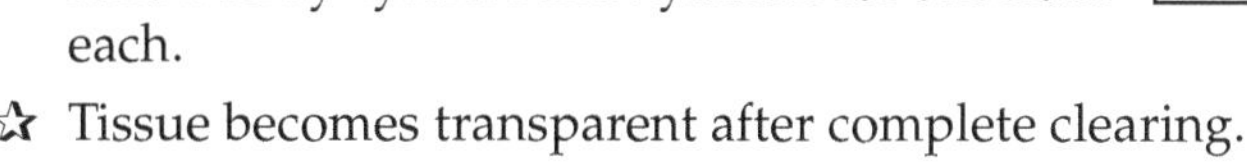

- ☆ Tissue becomes transparent after complete clearing.

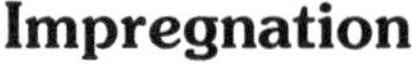

Impregnation

- ☆ Paraffin wax is used for the impregnation of tissue block.
- ☆ Paraffin wax is used in paraffin embedding bath at 60-62°C for liquefaction.
- ☆ At the time of transfer of tissue block from xylene II, the paraffin bath must be kept at 60-62°C, at this temp paraffin wax will be in liquid form and it will available for proper impregnation. Three changes are given in paraffin wax each of one hour.

Casting of Blocks

Methods of hardening the tissues for section cutting.

- Freezing
- Embedding in a hard material such at paraffin wax or gelatin.

- The blocks are formed in moulds using molten wax.
- The tissue are placed in moulds in various type of moulds like "L" shaped or ring shaped in such a way that desired surface should be downward on the base of mould.
- The sections are cut from this surface.
- The mould is filled with molten paraffin wax and then blocks are cooled at room temp or in cold water.

Trimming

- Blocks are removed from moulds and excess wax around mould is trimmed by knife or by rubbing on hot plate so that the tissue is exposed.
- It facilitates the side determination on which section is to be cut.

Section Cutting

- Microtome is being used for thin uniform tissue section.
- The various types of microtomes, rotary microtome, freezing microtome, sledge microtome and ultra microtome are available for this purpose.
- The block is attached to the holder of microtome in such a manner so that top and bottom of the block is parallel and horizontal to edge of knife.
- Usually the sections are cut at 4-6 µm thickness on rotator microtome using a plain edge knife. The knife should be sharp so that it cuts the desired thickness sections in the form of ribbon and does not damage to tissue.

Fixing of Sections to Slides

- Paraffin sections become compressed and creased. Sections are transferred from the cutting edge of microtome knife with the help of a spatula to a tissue flotation bath having warm water (40-50°C) for removal of creases and flatten the sections.
- Uniformly spread sections on water are then taken on clean glass slide coated with albumin-glycerin mixture in 1:1 ratio.
- The section slides are transferred in to incubator (40-50°C)minimum for 1 hour or overnight at 37°C to ensure drying of sections so that section become ready for staining.

Staining

Following procedure are being used for staining:

Paraffin Removal

Haematoxylin and Eosin staining
Nucleus - Blue
Cytoplasm and background - Pink

- ✰ Slides are slightly warmed in incubator or in sprit lamp and then placed in xylene jar for 10-15 min.
- ✰ Change the xylene with another fresh xylene after 10 to 15 min.

Rehydration

- ✰ Keep the slides in descending series of alcohol.
- ✰ First keep in mixture of xylene and absolute alcohol in 1:1 ratio for 5 min then place in absolute alcohol, 95 per cent, 90 per cent, 80 per cent, 70 per cent, 60 per cent ethanol for 5-6 min in each dilution.
- ✰ After that emerge into the water.

Cleaning of Slides

- ✰ Clean the slide from both the side with the help of muslin cloth.
- ✰ Wash the slide in running water for removal of extra sections and remnants of paraffin wax.

Hematoxylene Staining

- ✰ Keep the slides in hematoxylene for 10-15 min and wash in running tap water.
- ✰ Dip the slide in acid alcohol for few seconds and Wash the slide is tap water and place in ammonia water for few seconds.
- ✰ Again wash in running tap water to remove the ammonia.

Eosine Staining

Keep the slides in 2 per cent aqueous eosin for 2-5 min.

Dehydration

- ✰ Keep the slide in 70 per cent, 80 per cent, 90 per cent, 95 per cent and absolute ethanol for 5 min in each solution.
- ✰ Finally place in mixture of ethanol and xylene in 1:1 ratio for 5 min.

Cleaning

- ✰ Dips the slide in xylene and gives two changes at least for 10-15 min each.

Mounting

- ✰ DPX or Canada balsam is being used for mounting purpose.
- ✰ Keep the coverslips of desired size and shape on filter paper.
- ✰ One or two drops of mountant are place on coverslip.

- ☆ Slide placed on coverslip in such a way that the section touches the mountant.
- ☆ Press gently and lift the slide and remove the air bubble with the help of forceps.
- ☆ Now the slide is kept in horizontal position in tray for drying.

Cleaning and Labeling

- ☆ Slide cleaning is done after drying with the help of muslin cloth and xylene. Remove extra mount with a blade.
- ☆ Level the slide with a piece of paper and stick it on one corner with adhesive.
- ☆ At the time of examination histopathologist should put the name of organ, main changes in sections or disease condition with other remarks on this level.

Chapter 13

Examination of Biopsy and Morbid Material for Laboratory Diagnosis

Biopsy

Biopsy is a surgical procedure that involves removal of tissue from a living organism for disease diagnosis. Biopsies may be performed on almost all organs like breast, kidneys, liver, bone marrow, bone, skin, lung, lymph nodes, muscles, nerves, testes, thyroid, bladder, heart, neck, prostate etc.

Indications

- ☆ Diagnosing of abscess, tumors and cancers.
- ☆ Diagnosing of bone lesions which are not specifically identified through clinical and radiography.
- ☆ Monitor the inflammatory changes of unknown cause that persist for long periods.
- ☆ Diagnosing of autoimmune disorders.

Types of Biopsy

1. Cytology
2. Excisional biopsy
3. Incisional biopsy
4. Fine needle aspiration biopsy

Cytology

Cytology allows examination of individual cells, but cannot provide the histological features crucial for an accurate and definitive diagnosis. It is preliminary used for diagnostic screening procedure to monitor large tissue areas for dysplastic changes.

Advantages of Cytology

- ☆ Samples can be collected easily and quickly
- ☆ Prepared, stained and interpreted quickly
- ☆ Inexpensive
- ☆ Little or no risk to the animal

Cytology

Exfoliative cytology - Spontaneously shed cells in body fluids *e.g.*, Urine, CSF, Sputum, Effusions in body cavities (pleura, pericardium, peritoneum).

Abrasive cytology – Dislodges cells from body surfaces from body surfaces through Imprint Scraping, endoscopic brushing of mucosal surfaces, washing (lavage) of mucosal or serosal surfaces and Swab.

Fine needle aspiration cytology - Use of a needle and syringe to remove a sample of cells or contents of a lesion. The inability to withdraw fluid or air indicates that the lesion is probably solid.

Excisional Biopsy

Whole organ or a whole lump is removed (excised). These are less common now, since the development of fine needle aspiration. Some types of tumors (such as lymphoma, a cancer of the lymphocyte blood cells) have to be examined whole to allow an accurate diagnosis, so enlarged lymph nodes are good candidates for excisional biopsies. Some organs, such as the spleen, are dangerous to cut into without removing the whole organ, so excisional biopsies are preferred for these.

Incisional Biopsy

Only a representative portion of the lesion is removed surgically. If the lesion is large or has many differing characteristics, more than one area may require sampling. This type of biopsy is most commonly used for tumors of the soft tissues (muscle, fat, connective tissue) to distinguish benign conditions from malignant soft tissue tumors, called sarcomas.

Endoscopic Biopsy

This is probably the most commonly performed type of biopsy. It is done through a fiberoptic endoscope inserts into the gastrointestinal tract (alimentary tract).

Abrasive Cytology Procedures

1. Scrape the lesion repeatedly and firmly with the help of moistened tongue depressor or cytology brush.
2. Transfer the cells scrape material on a glass slide and make a thin smear over it.
3. Immerse the slide in a fixing solution.

4. Stained with any proper tissue staining solution (H and E stain) and examined under the microscope.

Fine Needle Aspiration Biopsy Procedures

1. Connect18-gauge needle to a 5 or 10 ml syringe and is insert into the center of the mass via a small hole in the lesion.
2. Positioned the tip of the needle in multiple directions to locate a potential fluid center.

Aspirate the Fluid Slowly in the Syringe

Lesion can be identifies base upon the consistency of fluid

- Straw-coloured fluid - Cystic lesion.
- Purulent exudates (pus) - Inflammatory or infectious process.

Incision Biopsy Procedure

1. Representative areas are biopsied in a wedge fashion.
2. Margins should extend into normal tissue on the deep surface.
3. Necrotic tissue should be avoided.
4. The sample should be taken from the edge of the lesion to include surrounding normal tissue
5. It should be deep enough to include underlying changes of the surface lesion.

Excisional Biopsy Procedure

1. An excisional biopsy implies the complete removal of the lesion.
2. A perimeter of normal tissue (2-3 mm) surrounding the lesion is included with the specimen.
3. Excisional biopsy should be performed on smaller lesions (less than 1 cm in diameter) that appear clinically benign.
4. Pigmented and vascular lesions should be removed, if possible, in their entirety. This avoids seeding of the melanin producing tumor cells into the wound site or in the case of a hemangioma, allows the clinician to address the feeder vessels.
5. Pigmented and vascular lesions should be removed, if possible, in their entirety. This avoids seeding of the melanin producing tumor cells into the wound site or in the case of a hemangioma, allows the clinician to address the feeder vessels.

Necropsy

Necropsy is systematic examination of an dead animal. It provides a simple consistent method to examine a carcass and its body organs. The procedures are

Sample Collected during Necropsy

Sl.No.	Name of Disease	Sick/lLive Animals	Dead Animals
Bacterial diseases			
1.	Haemorrhagic Septicemia	Fixed Smears from blood and throat swelling	Smears from heart blood and Liver. Heart blood in sterile bottle, lymph node and spleenon ice
2.	Black Quarter	Impression smears from affected muscle tissues and exudates from lesions on ice	Pieces of affected muscles on ice
3.	Anthrax	Flame fixed smears:From blood in cattle and sheep. From subcutaneous swelling in horse, swine and dogs	Swab of blood from ear vein for cultural examination or piece of ear in saline or without any preservative in sterile bottle on ice duly sealed.
4.	Enterotoxaemiaor lamb Dysentery		Contents of small intestine with or without chloroform separately on ice, Kidney and urine
5.	Brucellosis	Paired serum samples, Vaginal swabs in PBS in separate bottle on ice, Neat semen in sterile vial or semen straws on ice.	Paired serum samples, Vaginal swabs in PBS in separate bottle on ice, Neat semen in sterile vial or semen straws on ice.
6.	Compylobacteriosis	In males: Prepucial mucus/smegma/washing in specific media. In females: Vaginal mucus/lavage.	In females: Aborted foetus/placenta/stomach contents
7.	Johne'sDisease	Rectal pinch smears, bowl washing (at least 10 g preserved in 10 per cent neutral formal saline solution)	Terminal portion of ilium with ilio-caecal valve, mesenteric lymph gland in 10 per cent neutral formal saline solution.
8.	Glanders	Exudates from skin and lung lesions in vials on ice. Impression smears from exudates duly fixed	
9.	Tuberculosis	Cough material in sterile container from live animals, Sample of milk in sterile container	Smears from lesions fixed by heat, lymph glands, lung lesions in sterile containers for bacterial isolation in 50 per cent buffered glycerin
10.	Leptospirosis	Blood serum, Milk and urine about 20 ml in sterile vials byadding 1 drop of formalin	Pieces of liver, kidney in 10 per cent neutral formal saline solution
11.	Salmonellosis	Intestinal swab, heart blood, bile in sterile container on ice	
12.	Actinomycosis and Actinobacillosis	Smears from pus lesions, Pus in vial on ice	Formalin preserved materials from affected muscle.

Contd...

Contd...

Sl.No.	Name of Disease	Sick/lLive Animals	Dead Animals
13.	Listeriosis		Aborted foetus, brain, placenta and all internal organs in sterile vials on ice and 10 per cent neutral formal saline solution
14.	Mycoplasmosis/CCPP/ CBPP/COryza	Paired serum samples, swabs from lesions, nasal and vagina in PBS on ice.	Piece of lung preserved in 10 per cent formalin for histopathological examination and on ice
15.	Contagious Equine Metritis	Urogenital swabs from mare and stallion, paired serum samples	
16.	MycoticInfections	Deep Skin Scrappings in sterlie vials for fungal isolation.	
		Viral Diseases	
1.	Foot and Mouth Disease	Vescicular fluid from unruptured oral vesicles and epithelium from fresh lesions in 50 per cent GPB	Pieces of pancreas, heart and other organs on ice
2.	PPR	Eye, mouth, nasal, rectal swabs in PBS on Ice, Blood at the height of temperature in anticoagulent, Pre-scapular lymph node biopsy.	Lymphnodes, spleen pieces of intestine on ice, all other vital tissues on ice and 10 per cent formalin
3.	Rabies	Corneal swab	Half portion of brain in 50 per cent GPB and half in 10 per cent formalin
4.	Pock Diseases	Scabs in sterile container on ice/50 per cent GPB	Skin lesions in 10 per cent neutral formal saline separatel
5.	Infectious bovine Rhinotracheitis	Paired serum on ice, Swabs from vaginal and nasal lesions from suspected animals. From bulls neat semen sample on ice.	
6.	Classical Swine Fever	Paired serum	Spleen, lymph node and pancreas (10 to 15 g each) in 50 per cent GPB. Pieces of brain, lungs, intestines especially ileo- caecal region and kidney in 10 per cent neutral formal saline. For isolation do not put glycerine and send material on ice
7.	Blue Tongue	Blood at the height of temperature in heparin, paired sera samples	Spleen and lymph node on ice for virus isolation. All vital organs to be collected in 10 per cent neutral formal saline.

Contd...

Contd...

Sl.No.	Name of Disease	Sick/ILve Animals	Dead Animals
8.	Caprine Arthritis Encephalitis	Paired serum	Joint capsule, brain and lungs in 10 per cent formalin and on ice.
9.	Equine Influenza	Nasal swabs in VTM on ice and paired serum	Vital organs on ice and in 10 per cent formal saline.
10.	Equine Infectious Anaemia	Paired serum	All internal organs in 10 per cent neutral formal saline solution
11.	African Horse Sickness	Paired serum sample	Spleen, brain and lungs in 50 per cent buffered Glycerine and 10 per cent Formal saline separately
12.	Ranikhet Disease	Serum samples	Freshly dead/morbid bird on ice, pieces of liver, spleen, trachea, bronchi, lungs in 50 per cent buffered glycerine saline on ice and provetriculus in 10 per cent neutral formal saline solution.
13.	Marek's Disease	Paired serum, feather follicles from chest and neck region in transport medium	Portion of peripheral nerve, trachea, ovary, liver, kidney, spleen and skin in 10 per cent neutral formal saline solution.
14.	Avian Influenza	Cloacal, nasal Swabs Faecal content in VTM on ice	Dead Bird, All important vital organs in VTM on ice and in 10 per cent neutral formal saline
15.	Infectious Bursal Disease	Affected bird,Paired serum	Bursa of fabritious in transport medium, Kidney,spleen and bursa of fabritious in 10 per cent neutral formal saline solution.
16.	Lichee Heart Disease	Liver, spleen, bursa, kidney, heart on ice and in 10 per cent formalin	

Contd...

Contd...

Parasitic Diseases

Sl.No.	Name of Disease	Samples
1.	Babesiosis	Thin blood smears from early stage of disease taken from ear vein fixed with methanol
2.	Theileriosis	Biopsy smears from swollen lymph nodes fixed with methanol, blood smears from each case from ear vein fixed with methanol
3.	Anaplasmosis	Thin blood smears from early stage of disease taken from ear vein fixed with methanol
4.	Trichomoniasis	In females-vaginal and uterine discharge just before and after abortion In males- preputial washing in transport media
5.	Trypanaosomiasis/surra	Blood in anticoagulant on ice and fixed blood smears
6.	Gastrointestinal Parasites	Faecal sample in 10 per cent neutral Formal Saline solution and from dead animals' parasites for identification.
7.	Lungworm Infestations	Faecal sample in 10 per cent neutral Formal Saline solution. Nasal swabs in PBS or normal saline and infected lung tissues in formal saline
8.	Ectoparsitic Infestations	Deep skin scrapings in sterile vials.

particularly important where there are numbers of animals at risk or where disease prevalence is poorly documented in the species or animal group being investigated.

Types of Necropsy

Partial Necropsy

A partial necropsy may be performed depending on the size of the animal. Small animals should be partially necropsied and entirely fixed in formalin for further laboratory investigate.

Full Necropsy

Start with external examination of the animal body. Any external parasites and consider collection of these for identification. Any wounds, swellings, ulcers or other abnormalities and consider sampling into formalin.

Observations Procedure

- Signalmen – species, breed, sex, sexual status, age, colour
- History and clinical diagnosis
- Clinical pathology
- External appearance
- Body condition
- Mucous membranes
- Body orifices
- General conformation
- Superficial lesions (tumors, dermatitis, etc.)
- Hair coat
- Parasites
- Lips, gums, cheeks, teeth.

Chapter 14

Isolation of Bacteria from Clinical Specimens, Identification of Bacteria by Gram's Staining and Cultural/Biochemical Characteristics

Isolation of Bacteria from Clinical Specimens

Diagnostic bacteriology is concerned with the isolation and identification of bacteria in clinical sample. Most of clinical sample contain mixtures of the disease-producing bacteria and the host's normal flora rather than single bacterial type. Since accurate studies of a bacterial species are possible only through the use of pure cultures, it is necessary to isolate the pathogenic organisms from the sample through a reliable and rapid method.

Material Requires

- ☆ Flaming/Inoculating Loop: Used for making transfers of bacterial cultures
- ☆ Bunsen burner: Source for sterilization of loop
- ☆ Petri dish containing media: Nutrient source for bacteria
- ☆ The clinical specimens: Body fluid (blood, CSF) discharges (sputum, urine, feces).
- ☆ Luria Broth/nutrient broth: General type of media that allows all types of bacteria to grow
- ☆ Incubator
- ☆ Water bath

A colony is a large number of bacterial cells on solid medium, which is visible to the naked eye as a discrete entity. In pure culture one colony represent clone of one bacterial cell.

Methods of Inoculation

Streak Plate Method

A small droplet of culture or sample is spread over the surface of the medium with an inoculating loop or swab and then streaked over the surface according to the pattern that gradually thins out the sample and separates the cells.

Procedure

1. Sterilize the inoculum loop and place a loop-full culture/sample on the agar surface and make 3-4 parallel streaks across the surface without breaking it.
2. Flame the inoculation loop again and draw 3-4 parallel streaks across the first streak.
3. Repeat the streak 3-4 times across the previous streaks evenly.
4. Incubate at 37°C for 24-48 hrs.
5. Select the individual colony and inoculate on a slant for further characterization and preservation.

Pour Plate Method

The sample is diluted serially into a series of nutrient broth so as to dilute the number of cells sufficiently to obtain separate colonies when plating the small volumes of several diluted samples are mixed with liquid agar that has been cooled to 45°C and mixtures are poured immediately into sterile petri plates and are allowed to solidify. The number of cells in the tubes has ample space; each cell is fixed in place to grow into separate colonies. In this technique some of the colonies will develop deep in the medium itself and not on the surface.

Preservation methods of bacterial culture

- ✰ Subculture,
- ✰ Sterile mineral oil on slant culture, refrigerator at 4° to 10°C,
- ✰ Stab inoculate,
- ✰ Lyophilization (freeze-drying).

Spread Plate Method

A small volume of liquid/diluted sample is pipetted on the surface of the medium and spread evenly by a sterile spreading L shaped glass rod. Cells are pushed into separate areas on the surface so that they can form individual colonies.

Identification of Bacteria

Direct Microscopic Examination

The examination of wet mounts of unstained materials by phase contrast or dark field microscopy is useful for demonstrating motility, spirochaetes and endospores.

Wet Mount Slide

It is the simplest way to see the isolated bacteria. A few loopfuls of the organism place on a clean slide and cover it with a cover glass. In addition to being able to determine the presence or absence of motility, this method is useful in determining cellular shape (rod, coccus, or spiral) and arrangement (irregular clusters, packets, pairs, or long chains).

Hanging Drop Slide

It is useful in observing the general shape of living bacteria and their arrangement as such. A drop of bacterial culture put on the cover glass and places it on the concave depression of slide. In this position cover glass holds a drop of the suspension in the center of cavity. See the slide under the microscope. Since the drop lies within an enclosed glass chamber, drying out occurs very slowly. Vaseline around the edge of the cover slip can also be applied to prevent drying.

Stains and Staining Procedure of Bacteria

The basic principle of staining is to visualize bacteria by increasing contrast. They can be stained by certain dyes *e.g.* aqueous methylene blue, Loffler's alkaline methylene blue and dilute carbol fuschin. Differential staining involve use of more than one dye and helps in differentiation of bacteria in two groups for *e.g.* Gram's Staining and Acid fast staining.

> **Fixation of bacterial smear**
>
> ✰ Kills the bacteria by denaturing the protein
>
> ✰ Adhere the bacterial smear to the slide.
>
> ✰ Allows diffusion of stain into the cytoplasm.

Preparation of Bacterial Smear

1. Take a slide and make it free from dirt, moisture and grease by using muslin cloth and flame.
2. Place a drop of normal saline on the centre of slide with the help of sterile platinum loop.
3. Sterilize the platinum loop by heating it red hot with Bunsen burner and allows cooling on media plate in the area not having no growth. Touch the loop to a separate or isolated colony.
4. Mix with normal saline and spread thoroughly on the slide.
5. Air dry and fix it gently over the flame.

> **Common method of fixation is gentle heating and passing the slide several times through the hot portion of the flame of a Bunsen burner of dry slide.**

Gram's Staining

Principle

Bacterial cells take the stain of primary dye crystal violet. Gram's iodine act as mordent and form large crystals with primary dye that are trapped by peptidoglygan layer in cell wall. The peptidoglygan layer in Gram positive cell wall in thicker (20-80 nm) than Gram negative cells (8-10 nm) and contain lesser lipid. Gram positive bacteria contain magnesium ribonucleoprotein in their cell wall which forms complex with

> In **negative, indirect,** or **background staining** acidic stain such as nigrosin, India ink, or eosin, do not penetrate the bacterial cells due to repulsion between the negative charge of the stains and the negatively charged bacterial wall and produce a dark background in which bacteria appear as unstained cells with a clear area around them.

crystal violet and Gram's iodine are resistant to decolorize and do not take the counter stain. The Gram negative bacteria dye do not form complex in absence of magnesium ribonucleoprotein and decolouriser dissolves the lipid in the outer membrane and removes dye from the cells and take the counter stain.

Procedure

1. Prepare a thin bacterial smear, air dry and fix.
2. Place the slide on crystal violet stain for 2 min.
3. Wash with tap water.
4. Add Gram's iodine for 1 minute and wash with tap water.
5. Decolourize with (95 per cent) alcohol (ethanol) or with a mixture of alcohol and acetone and do not wash with tap water.
6. Blot dry.
7. Counter stain with safranin or dilute carbol fuschin for 15 to 20 second.
8. Wash with tap water, blot dry and examine under oil emersion.

Interpretation

Gram Positive: Blue or violet colour organism.

Gram negative: Pink or red colour organism.

Acid Fast Staining/Ziehl- Neilson's Staining

Principle

High lipid contents (Mycolic acid) in the cell wall mycobacterium resist staining. The stain is facilitated by heat. Once stained, they retain the colour of dye and do not decolourize by suitable decolourizer (dilute acid).

> **Kinyoun** procedure also stain the acid fast bacteria without heating the slide so called **cold staining** procedure.

Stains

Primary stain - Carbol fuschin

Decolourizer - Acid alcohol (3 per cent hydrochloric acid in 95 per cent ethyl alcohol)

Counter stain - Methylene blue

Procedure

1. Prepare the smear of mycobacterium culture air dry and fixed it.
2. Stain the smear with Ziehl Neilson carbol fuschin and heat the slide on burner or sprit lamp till the steam appears.
3. Continue intermittent heating for 3-5 minutes; avoid drying the stain during the process.
4. Wash the smear with tap water after cooling.

5. Decolorize the smear with acid alcohol for 20-30 seconds until the smear is faint or colourless.
6. Counter stain the smear with methylene blue for 1 minute.
7. Wash the slide with water, air dry the smear and observe under oil immersion.

Interpretations

Red colour organism -Acid fast

Blue colour organism- Non acid fast.

Capsule Staining

Principle

Capsule present in the outer most covering of the bacteria. The presence of capsule is considered as the indication of the virulence and pathogenicity. It is antigenic in nature and made up to polysaccharide except in *B. anthracis* where it is polypeptide in nature. The capsule can be stained by Hiss copper surface method.

Procedure

1. Make smear in serum, air dry and fix it by gentle heat.
2. Apply Gentian violet stain and heat gently until steam rises.
3. Allow the dyes to act for 15-20 seconds.
4. Wash the dye with 20 per cent $CuSO_4$ solution.
5. Do not wash with water, blot dry and examine under oil immersion.

Interpretation

Capsule appears as a blue halo around the dark purple cell body against a faint purple back ground.

Spore Staining

Principle

Some bacteria *e.g.* Clostridium produces spores under unfavorable condition. The shape and position of these spores, is very useful in the species characterization of bacteria. These spores are difficult to stain, but once stained they are difficult to decolorize. Modified Zeihl Neilson method of staining used to stain the spore.

Procedure

1. Make a smear and fixed over the flame.
2. Flood the smear with conc. Carbol fuschin and steam for 3-4 minutes.

> Schaeffer-Fulton method can also be used for staining of endospore. **Malachite green** is used for staining which give green colour to the endospore.

3. Wash the slide with tap water.
4. Decolorizes smear with 0.5 per cent sulfuric acid.
5. Wash with tap water.
6. Counter stain with Loffler's alkaline methylene blue for 2 minutes.
7. Spores will appear Red while the vegetative cells appear blue.

Morphological Identification of Bacterial Isolates

On the basis of staining and morphology the isolates may be identified on following points

Morphological Characteristics

> **Blood Agar** is both a differential medium and an enriched one. It distinguishes between hemolytic and nonhemolytic bacteria.

1. **Shape**: Spherical or Cocci, coccobacillary, short or long rods, filamentous, comma-shaped, curved or spherical forms.
2. **Size**: spherical are measured in diameter and rod shaped in length and breadth. Measurement is expressed in microns (μ) and is done with the help of microscope. This process is called as micrometry.
3. **Sides**: straight, concave, bulging, parallel or irregular.
4. **Ends**: Round, Pointed, truncate or concave.
5. **Axis**: Straight or curved.
6. **Arrangement**: Single, in pairs, in groups of four or eight, in grape- like clusters, in a long chain, or scattered irregularly, may be in bundles, angular arrangements or in Chinese letters (Palisade arrangement).
7. **Pleomorphism**: Bacteria present in the given smear may differ from their typical shape and size. Older cultures may differ greatly from their typical forms. Variations may be in shape, size, and staining behavior.
8. **Capsule**: May or may not be present. When present, it may be thin or thick or slime layer may be present. This can only be revealed only by special staining.
9. **Flagella**: Bacteria may be atrichous, monotrichochous, amphitrichous, lophotrichous or peritrichous.
10. **Motility**: Present or absent. This should be tested in young broth culture. Motility should be confused with Brownian or molecular movement which is a to and fro motion without change in position.
11. **Endospores**: Some species are sporulated. Spores may be spherical or oval. The location of the spore may be central, sub-terminal or terminal in the cell and may not bulge the bacteria. Mature spores do not stain with Gram's Method; they can be stained with modified Zeihl- Neilson method.

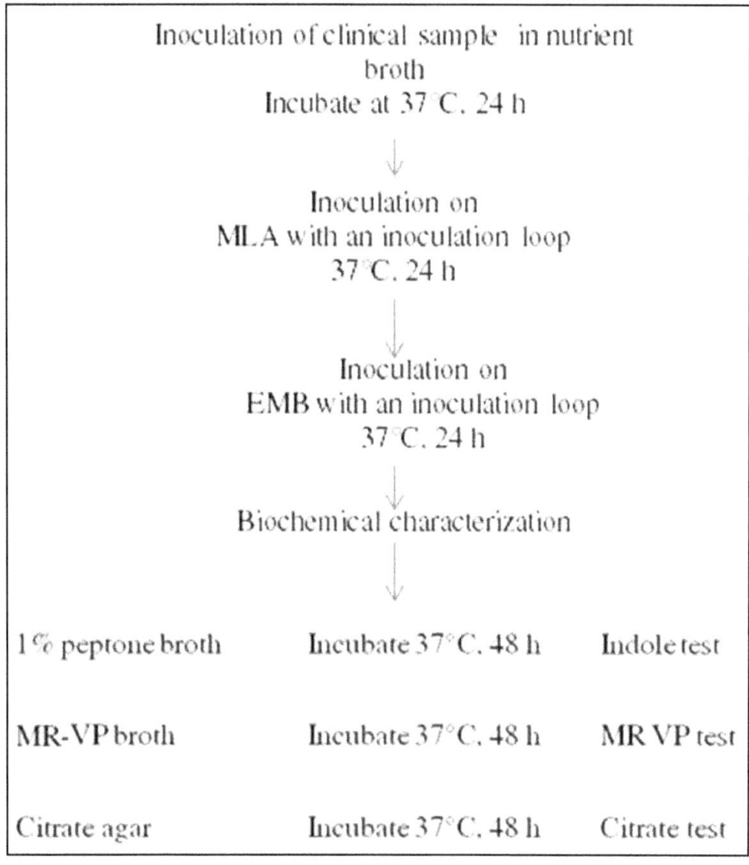

Steps for the Isolations *E. coli* from Clinical Sample.

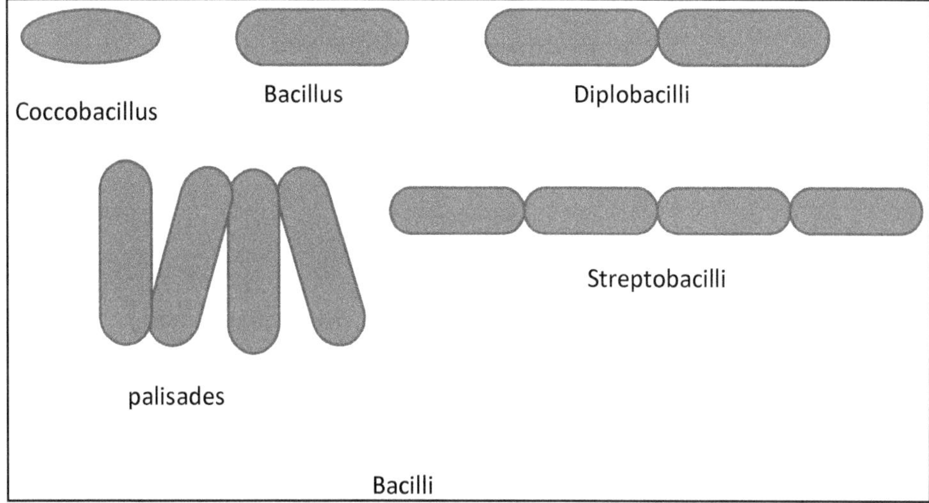

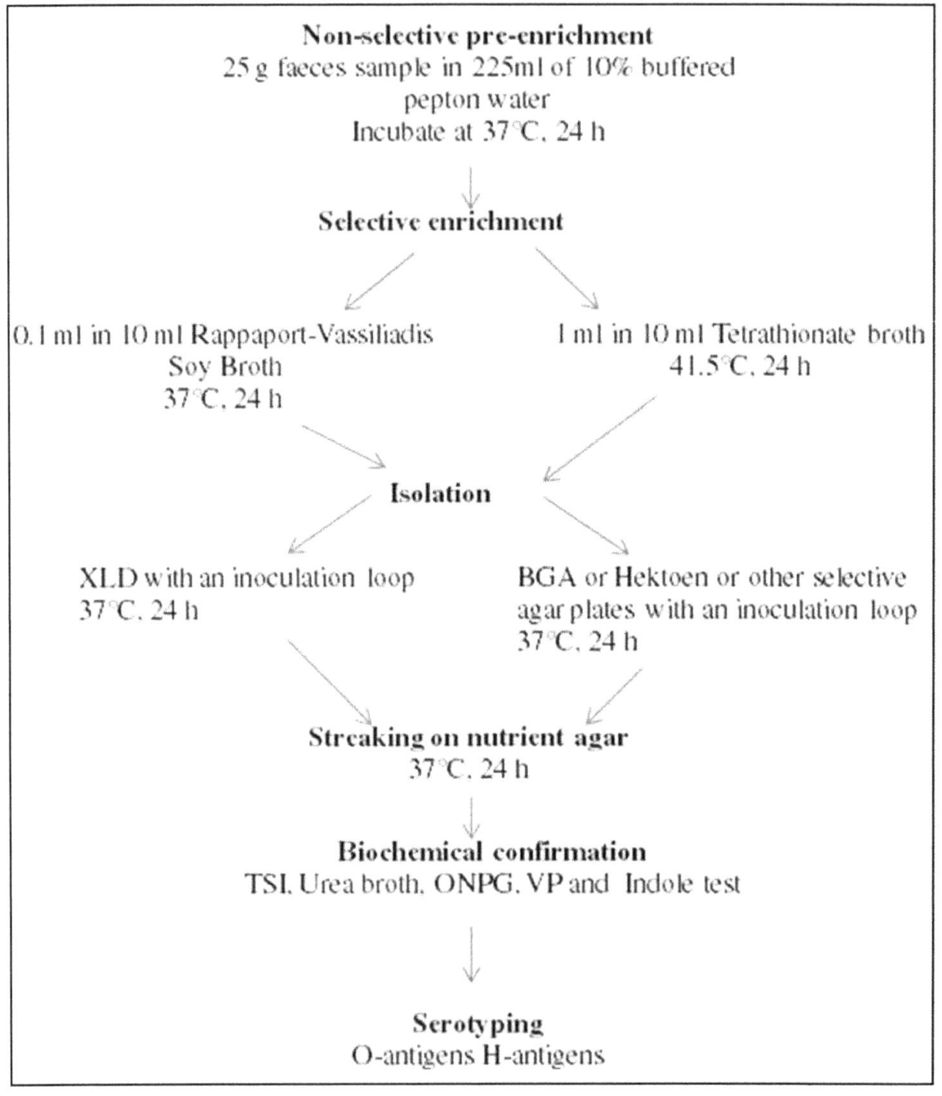

Step for the Isolations *Salmonella* spp. from Poultry Faeces

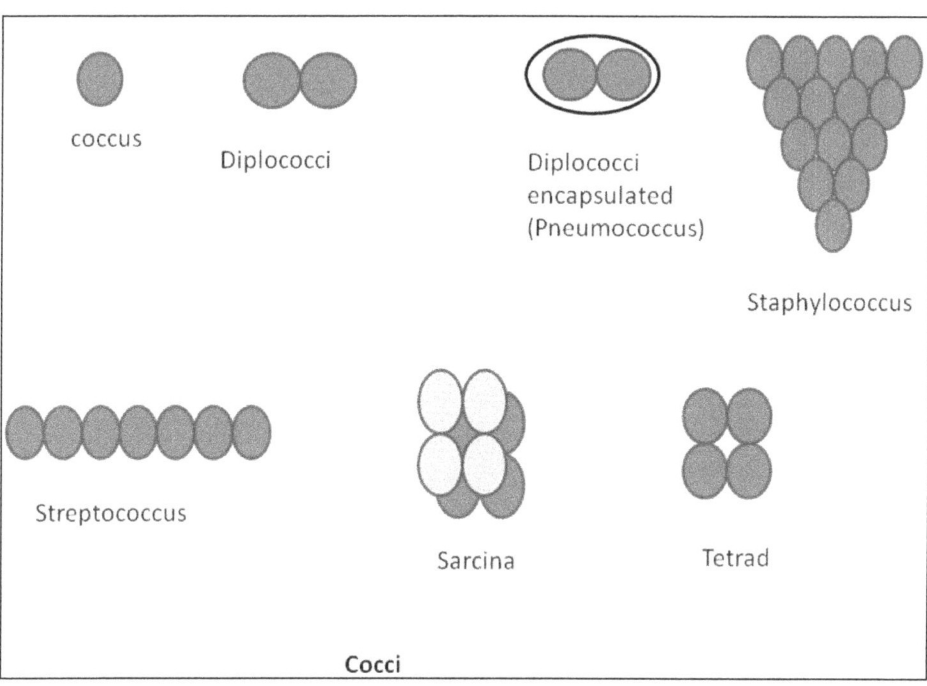

Cocci

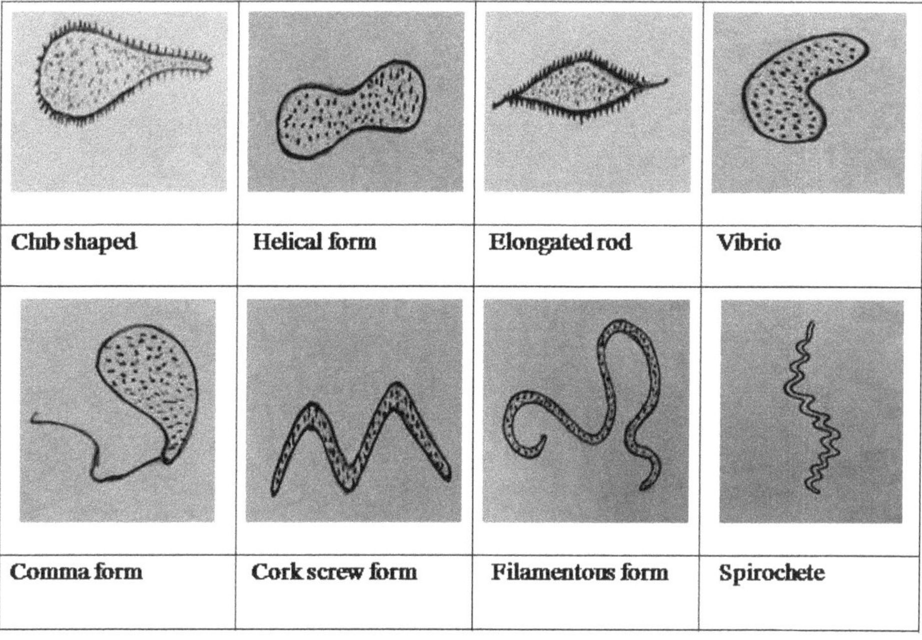

Other bacteria

Staining Reaction: Reaction of Gram's or Zeihl- Neilson's stain should be noted. The staining may be uniform, unipolar, and bipolar beaded or there may be presence or absence of metachromatic granules. Some cells may show deeper colour than others.

Cultural Identification of Bacterial Isolates

Study of cultural characteristics is essential for identification of bacteria. Routine examination of which may be studied under following steps:

Surface Colonies on Solid Media

1. Shape: Round, irregular, spindle, rhizoid (irregularly branched)
2. Size: in mm.
3. Elevation: Flat, raised, convex, umbonate (convex with central knob)
4. Margins: Entire, undulate (wavy), lobate (with alternate lobes and sinuses). Crenated, erose (irregularly toothed), curled (like curly hairs with parallel filaments) filamentous.
5. Surface: Smooth, rough, ringed, papillate, granular.
6. Opacity: Opaque, translucent, transparent.
7. Consistency: Butyrous, friable, viscid (sticky).
8. Emulsifiability: Easy, difficult and homogenous or granular suspension.

Growth on Agar Slant

1. Amount of Growth: Scanty, moderate, abundant.
2. Form of Growth: Filiform (edges may be entire, undulate or erose), spreading rhizoid.
3. Growth in stab culture:
4. Amount of growth: Scanty, moderate, abundant.
5. Form of Growth: Filiform (edges may be entire the appearance of beads), papillate, arborescent (branched).
6. Surface growth: Absent/present, colouration.
7. Liquefaction (in case of gelatin stab): Crateriform (like a cup), napiform (like a turnip), saccateform (tubular), influndibuli form (like a funnel), stratiform (forming a layer) inverted fir like tree.

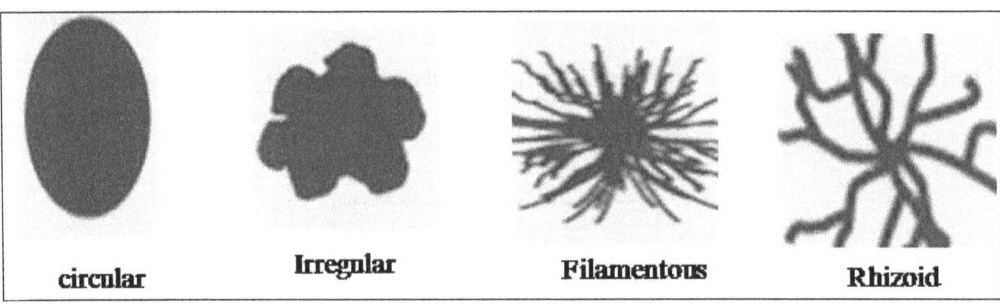

8. Growth in liquid medium
9. Amount of Growth: Scanty, moderate, abundant.
10. Surface growth: Absent/present, ring, pellicle (thin, thick, smooth or granular).
11. Deposit: Absent/present (slight, moderate, abundant, powdery, granular or viscid)
12. Turbidity: Absent/present
13. Odour: Absent/present

a. Biochemical Tests

Coagulase Test

Coagulase is an enzyme produced by some bacteria that converts (soluble) fibrinogen in plasma to (insoluble) fibrin. *Staphylococcus aureus* produces two forms of coagulase, bound and free. Coagulase test is used to differentiate *Staphylococcus aureus* (positive) from Coagulase Negative Staphylococcus (CONS). Slide coagulase test is done to detect bound coagulase or clumping factor. Tube coagulase test is done to detect free coagulase.

Slide Coagulase Test

1. Place a drop of plasma on clean grease free and dry glass slide.
2. Place a drop of distilled water for negative control.
3. Take a loop full of isolated colony and mixed with plasma.
4. Shake the slide gently for 5 to 10 seconds and observe for clumping (coagulation).

Tube Coagulase Test

1. Take 0.5 ml of plasma from horse, rabbit or man
2. Suspend a loop full of isolated colony in it.
3. Incubate this tube at 37°C.
4. After 4 h read the test. In case of negative result, continue with the incubation.
5. Final read perform after 24 h.

Interpretations

Positive reaction: Clot formation

Negative reaction: No clot formation or if the coagulate is dissolved again upon stirring.

Catalase Test

Principal

Catalase test is used to identify the many aerobic bacteria and most of those which are facultative anaerobic produce the enzyme Catalase. Catalase enzyme detoxifies hydrogen peroxide (H_2O_2) by breaking it in to H_2O and O_2 (gas), which is formed from superoxide radical by superoxide dismutase.

$$2\,H_2O_2 \rightarrow 2\,H_2O + O_2$$

Obligate anaerobic bacteria lack superoxide dismutase and catalase

Slide Method

1. Take a clean glass slide and labeled place a small drop of normal saline on two areas as "test" and "control".
2. Pick up a small amount of the culture from the nutrient agar slant or Petri plate.
3. Emulsify it on each drop to make a smooth suspension.
4. Place one drop of hydrogen peroxide over the test smear.
5. Do not put anything in the other drop that serves as control.
6. Observe the fluid over the smears for the appearance of gas bubbles.

Interpretations

Positive test: Bubbles formation due to production of oxygen gas.

Negative test: No gas formation.

Applications

To distinguish between catalase positive *Staphylococcus* spp. and catalase negative *Streptococcus* spp.

Citrate Test (Simmon's Citrate Agar Test)

Citrate test is performing to show the capability of bacterium to utilize citrate as the only carbon source. The enzyme citrase hydrolyzes citrate into oxaloacetic acid and acetic acid and finally formation of pyruvic acid and CO_2 occurs from the hydrolysis of oxaloacetic acid. If CO_2 is produced, it reacts with components of the medium to produce an alkaline compound (*e.g.* Na_2CO_3). The alkaline pH turns the pH indicator (bromthymol blue) from green to blue.

Procedure

1. Small amount of bacteria is inoculated in a "Simmons citrate tube" containing citrate medium.
2. Incubate this tube in incubator at 30-37°C for 24-48 h.

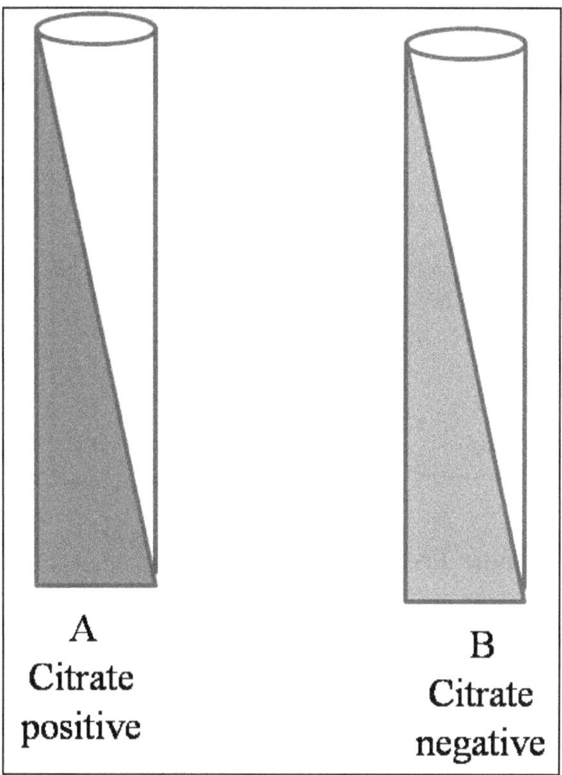

Interpretations

Positive test: Colour change to blue from green

Negative test: No colour change (still green colour).

Applications

- ☆ To differentiate members of Enterobacteriaceae.
- ☆ Bacterium *Klebsiella pneumoniae* and *Proteus mirabilis* are citrate positive organisms and *Escherichia coli* and *Shigella dysenteriae* are citrate negative.

Indole Test

Some bacteria produce tryptophanase enzyme that can hydrolyze the amino acid tryptophan to indole, pyruvic acid and ammonia. p-dimethylaminobenzaldehyde is present in Kovác's reagent which reacts with indole and forms a red complex.

Procedure

1. Suspend a colony from a pure culture of the bacterium into a tryptophan medium.

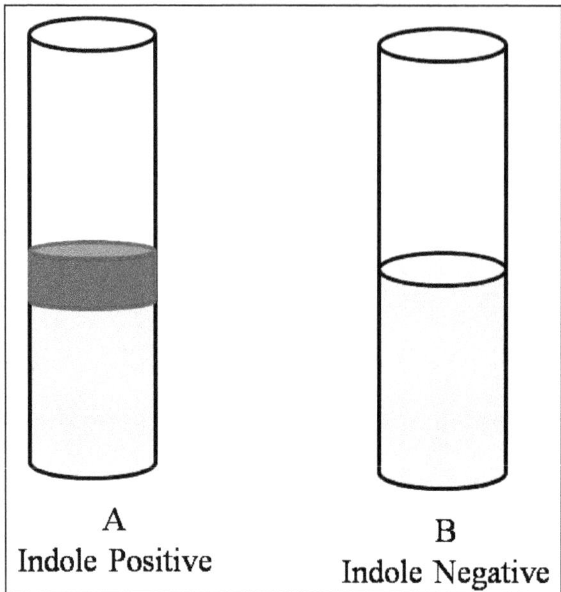

2. Incubate the tube in incubator at 37°C for 20-28 h.
3. Add a few drops of Kovác's reagent.

Interpretations

Positive test: Colour change to cerise red.

Negative test: No colour change (remain pale yellow).

Applications

- ✰ Confirmation of suspected *E. coli*-strains.
- ✰ Typing (species determination) of *Brachyspira* spp. in combination with other tests.

Methyl-Red Test

Some bacteria perform mixed acid fermentation when supplied glucose. Large amounts of acid produced significant decrease the pH of the medium below 4.4. Change in pH can be visualized by using pH indicator, methyl red (p dimethylaminoaeobenzene-O-carboxylic acid), which is yellow above pH 5.1 and red at pH 4.4.

Procedure

1. Take two MR-VP broths one for test and other for control.
2. Using aseptic conditions inoculate bacteria in one broth and leave the other broth without inoculation (control).
3. Place these tubes into the 35-37°C in incubator. This test is properly interpreted after 24 hours.

4. Obtain broths from the incubator and add a few drop of Methyl Red to each broth.
5. Within few minute observe the colour.

Interpretations

Positive test: Medium turns red.

Negative test: Culture medium remains yellow.

Applications

- ✫ Used to differentiate among the Gram-Negative bacilli in the family Enterobacteriaceae.
- ✫ MR Possitive: *Escherichia coli* and *Proteus vulgaris*.
- ✫ MR Negative: *Serratia marcescens* and *Enterobacter aerogenes*.

> Gases produced during the fermentation process within the liquid culture medium can be detected by using a small, inverted tube, called a **Durham tube**.

Voges-Proskauer (VP) Test

Some bacterium shows butanediol fermentation and can split glucose to acetoin via pyruvat and further to 2,3-butanediol.

2 pyruvate + NADH $\rightarrow$ 2CO_2 + 2,3-butanediol.

Acetoin converted into 2,3-butanedione (diacetyl) in presence of KOH (potassium hydroxide) which react with alpha-naphtol and forms a pink/red complex.

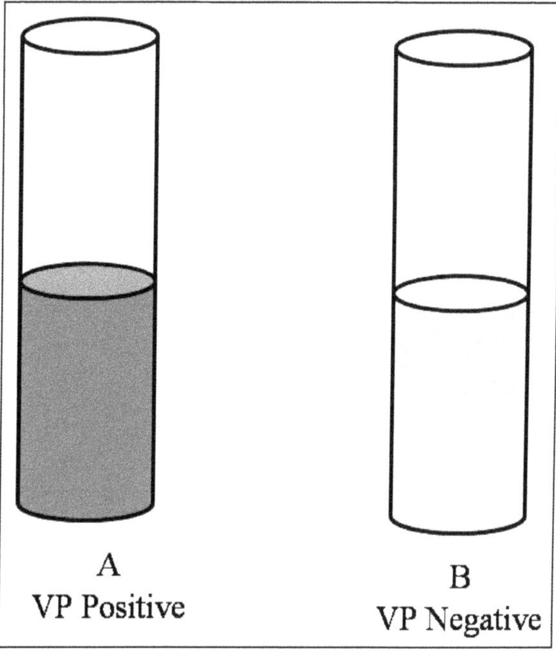

VP Reagent

1. Alpha-naphthol (VP reagent- I)
2. Potassium hydroxide (VP reagent-II)

Procedure

1. Suspend one colony from the pure culture, which is to be investigated, in VP/MR medium.
2. Incubate the tube in incubator at 30-37°C for 24-48 h.
3. Add 0.2 ml of 40 per cent KOH and then 0.6 ml of alpha-naphtol solution.

Interpretations

Positive test: Colour change to pink.

Negative test: No colour change.

Applications

- ☆ Tests for evidence of an enteric bacterium.
- ☆ VP positive: *Enterobacter, Klebsiella, Serratia marcescens.*
- ☆ VP negative: *Salmonella, Shigella, Yersinia, Edwardsiella, Citrobacter.*

CAMP Test (Christie, Atkins, and Munch-Petersen test)

CAMP factor is a diffusible protein produced by β-streptococci (group B) that complete haemolysis area formed by β-haemolysin from *Staphylococcus aureus.* Beta-haemolysin and CAMP factor interact with each other and produce synergistic haemolysis on blood agar plate.

Procedure

1. Make a single line streak of *Staphylococcus aureus* (produce beta-haemolysin) on blood agar plate
2. Inoculate a streak of beta-haemolytic *Streptococcus* perpendicular to the staphylococcal streak without intersecting it.
3. Streaks should be in such a way that the growth of two organism will not touch each other after incubation.
4. Streptococcal strain of group A and B should be similarly inoculated on the same plate as negatively and positively control respectively.
5. Plate should be incubating at 35°C in ambient air for 18-24 hours.

Interpretations

Complete hemolysis: CAMP factor producing streptococcus present.

Applications: To identify *Streptococcus agalactiaea* and *Listeria* spp.

Oxidase Test

Principal

The oxidase test is used to identify bacteria that produce cytochrome c oxidase, an enzyme of the bacterial electron transport chain. When present, the cytochrome c oxidase oxidizes the reagent (tetramethyl-p-phenylenediamine) to (indophenols) purple color end product. When the enzyme is not present, the reagent remains reduced and is colourless.

Reagent

1 per cent tetramethyl-p-phenylenediamine dihydrochloride.

Procedure

1. Apply two drops of the oxidase reagent after immediate opening of ampoule of oxidase reagent, onto a piece of filter paper.
2. Transfer bacteria from one colony with a platinum loop onto the spot with the oxidase reagent.
3. The colonies should have been incubated in incubator at the appropriate temperature for 18-24 hour.

Interpretations

Positive test: Dark blue-purple colour change within 10-30 sec.

Negative test: No colour change or colour change after more than 30 sec

Applications

- ✰ To identify members of the family Enterobacteriaceae
- ✰ Oxidase positive: Family Pseudomonadaceae, genus *Aeromonas* and *Campylobacte*
- ✰ Oxidase negative: Family Enterobacteriaceae (except genus *Plesiomonas*)

Urease Test

Ureas enzyme present in some bacteria which hydrolyzing urea in to ammonia and carbon di oxide. Ammonia increases the pH of medium due to weak base and medium turns alkaline.

Requirements

- ✰ Any urea medium, agar or broth
- ✰ Phenol red indicator

Procedure

1. Take a loop full of isolated colony and streak on the surface of a urea agar slant.
2. Leave the cap on loosely and incubate the test tube at 37°C for 48 hours to 7 days.

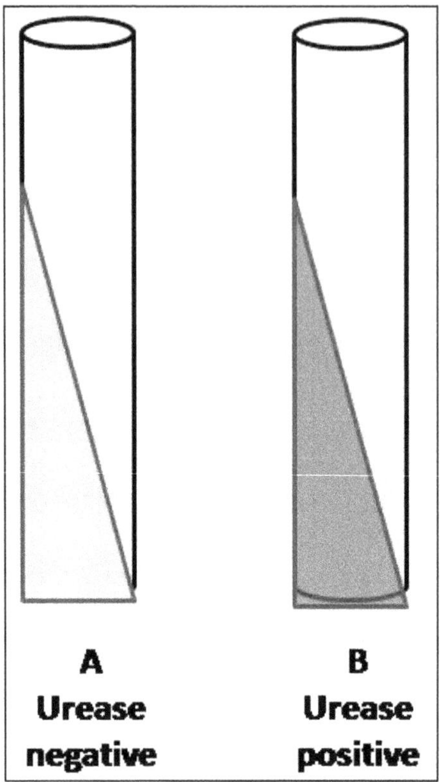

Interpretations

Positive: Colour changes red from yellow.

Negative: No colour change.

Applications

- ☆ Used to distinguish the genus *Proteus* from other enteric bacteria.

Chapter 15

Antibiogram-Drug Sensitivity and Rationale for Therapy

The antibacterial sensitivity test used to perform for the selecting specific antibiotics or when animal do not respond to the antibiotic treatment. Now antibiotic resistant in bacteria is common phenomenon. One of the reseaon is extensive and indiscriminate use of antibiotics in animals. Therefore, it is very necessary to carry out sensitivity test before the start of medication.

Modified Kirby-Beaur Method

It is commonly used for drug sensitivity test. The test is based on diffusion of drug from impregnated disc to agar medium when it came in contact with the agar surface. The growth of the organism is inhibited on agar media around the disc till the concentration of drug is below the critical level. The diameter of the resulting zone is considered proportional to the degree of susceptibility and allows to categories the organism into susceptible (S), intermediate (I), or resistant (R) when comparing with international guideline tables.

Materials

Mueller-Hinton agar plates, Antibiotics discs, Forceps, Sterile cotton swab, Broth media, Bacterial culture.

Procedure

1. Dip the sterile swab into the broth culture of the bacteria (approximately 1.5 X 10^8 CFU/ml).
2. Streak the swab over the entire surface of the fresh sterile Mueller-Hinton agar and allow the plate to stand for 5-10 minutes.
3. Place the antibiotics discs on the surface of agar with the help of sterilized forceps or an antibiotic disc dispenser, approximately at a distance of 24 mm. Generally up to 12 disks can be applied to a 150 mm diameter plate or up to 5 disks on a 100 mm plate.

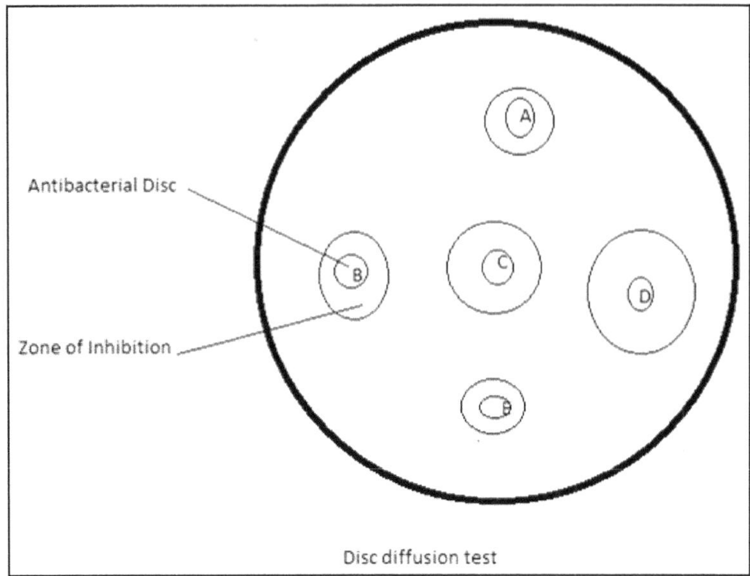

Disc diffusion test

4. Incubate the inoculated plate at 37°C for 24 hours.
5. Measure the zone of inhibition in mm.

Antibiogram Reading

- Diagonally measure the clear zones through the disc from the back of the plate using mm ruler or caliper.
- If the plates are not sufficiently grown, read again after 48 h incubation.
- If zones of inhibition produced by adjacent discs overlap to the extent that two measurements at right angles cannot be made, the zones around these discs should not be recorded.
- Use reflected light for Enterobacteriaceae, such as *E. coli*, other gram-negative bacilli, staphylococci, and enterococci (except for oxacillin and vancomycin).
- Use transmitted light when measuring zones for: *Staphylococci* with oxacillin *Enterococci* with vancomycin.

Interpretations

An interpretation of the sensitivity/resistance of the drug are made by composition of the zones of inhibition standard table and results are noted as follows:

Interpretation	*Zone*
Susceptible	Wider Zone of Inhibition
Intermediate	Moderate zone
Resistant	Very narrow or no zone

Precautions

- ✰ Press each disk down firmly to ensure complete level contact with the agar.
- ✰ Do not use disks beyond their expiration date.
- ✰ Do not store disks in a frost-free freezer.
- ✰ Do not relocate a disk once it has touched the agar surface.
- ✰ Invert and incubate plates with agar side up.

Rational Therapy

Now days, Clinical practice of human and veterinary medicine throughout the world involves use of a large number of antimicrobial drugs and non rational use of antimicrobial is common in day to day medical and veterinary practices. Prescribing drug without prompt diagnosis and microbial identification may provoke adverse effect of drug in body. These effects can be minimize by specific diagnosis and use of effectives antibiotic combinations which are useful in treating serious infections (mixed bacterial infections) and resistance infection.

Antibiotic resistant bacteria

- ✰ Methicillin-resistant *Staphylococcus aureus* (MRSA),
- ✰ Vancomycin-resistant *Enterococcus* (VRE)
- ✰ Multi-drug-resistant *Mycobacterium tuberculosis* (MDR-TB)
- ✰ Extensively drug-resistant *Mycobacterium tuberculosis* (XDR-TB)
- ✰ *Klebsiella pneumoniae* carbapenemase-producing bacteria (KPC)

It is based on selection of an appropriate antimicrobial agent and course of treatment that will inhibit or destroy the specific pathogens without compromising the animal's body system. Prime aim of rational therapy is to kill or eliminate the causative pathogen so that the host can recover without relapse and emergence of microbial resistance and drug-induced toxicity.

Principal of Rational Use of Antimicrobial

1. **Pathogen identification and characterization:** If first choice of antimicrobials treatment did not responded then select second choice of antimicrobial based upon identification and characterizing of organism including antimicrobial susceptibility.

Superbug is the bacteria having resistant to many drug.

NewDelhimetallo-beta-lactamaseand ***Klebsiellapneumoniaecarbapenemase*** producing gene present in superbug.

2. **Selection and combination of drug:** Among the susceptible drugs, one that is more likely to penetrate the infected tissue and suitable for host sex, species and breed should be chosen. A combination of drugs can also be used to potential the effect and reduce toxicity in animals.

3. **Dosing regimen:** The dosing regimen must be individualized to assure that the drug reaches the site at effective concentrations without harming the animals. Short-term therapy at high doses and short intervals should be sufficient to kill the infecting microbe. Longer duration therapy at lower concentrations should avoid as it might be facilitate resistance.
4. **Supportive therapy:** Specific and appropriate supportive or adjunctive therapy that enhances the animal's immunity and support the primary treatment to overcome the infection and associated disease conditions should use.

Common Point to be Consider before Use of Antimicrobials

- ✰ Veterinarian should have a working knowledge of commonly used antimicrobials.
- ✰ A narrow-spectrum antimicrobial should be chosen first.
- ✰ First-choice antimicrobials would comprise agents appropriate for initial treatment, not necessarily based on culture and sensitivity information.
- ✰ Second-choice antimicrobials should be prescribed based on culture and sensitivity data, provided that no first-choice agents are appropriate
- ✰ Have a good idea of the likely pathogen involved in infection.
- ✰ Ability to make a choice based on results from culture and sensitivity tests.
- ✰ Prophylactic use antimicrobial should be avoided.
- ✰ Correct dose, dose frequency and duration of treatment should be used.
- ✰ Use of too much or too little antimicrobial is avoided as it leads to development resistance.
- ✰ Avoid giving drugs in feed or in water as sub-therapeutic dosing is more comman in this practices.
- ✰ Time- and concentration-dependent killing should be taken into consideration.
- ✰ Avoid use of human use drugs in food animals.

Chapter 16

Diagnosis of Disease by Applying Tests like Agar Gel Precipitation Test, Enzyme Linked Immuno Sorbent Assay, Dot Immune Assay, Tube Agglutination Test, Plate/Slide Agglutination Test etc.

Agar Gel Precipitation Test

Agar gel precipitation test is qualitative method to detect the presence of antigen in sample or antibody in serum. This technique is described by Oudin and Ouchterlony, also called as Ouchterlony test or Double immunodiffusion test

Principle

The passive diffusion of soluble antigens and/or antibodies toward each other leads to their precipitation in a gel matrix which forms opaque precipitation line. It is highly specific and very sensitive for the detection of antigen.

Materials

1 per cent Agarose, Test antigen/Test serum, Positive serum, Negative serum, Negative antigen, Gel cutter - 4mm diameter, Petridish, Microscopic glass slide, Sodium Chloride, Micropipette.

Procedure

1. Prepare 1 per cent agarose by adding 1 g of agarose, 0.89 g of sodium chloride in 100 ml of distilled water and heating the mixture slowly to boiling point (Poultry 8 per cent sodium chloride is used).

2. Pour 4-5 ml of agarose on the clean slide when it cooled to 50°C to get a gel thickness of 2 to 2.5 mm.
3. Left the slide for 15- 20 minute to solidify the agarose.
4. Cut the 4 mm diameter well in the agrose with the help of well cutter. Keep the distance between two well 4 to 6 mm. There should be central well and 4-6 outer well around it.
5. Remove the agarose gel from wells with the help of needle.
6. Fill one drop of 0.1 per cent agarose in the bottom of each wells.
7. If antigen is to be detected then fill the known serum in the central wells and test samples in peripheral wells with help of micro pipette.
8. It is always desirable to have a positive control along with the test sample.
9. Place the slide in humid chamber (large petridish with wet filter paper) and incubat at 37 C for 24 hour.

Staining

Visibility and sensitivity of AGID can be increased by staining the gels with coomassie brilliant blue or amido black.

Procedure

1. Keep the slide overnight in sodium chloride (0.15 M) solution for the removal of non precipitating proteins and then placed in distilled water for 2 hours.
2. Dry the gels at room temp or in incubator at 37°C. Before drying, a drop of agar is placed in the well to prevent the cracking of wells on drying.
3. Stain it in 1 per cent Amido black, prepared in 7 per cent acetic acid for 5 min.
4. Destain the slide in solution of methanol: glacial acetic acid: distilled water (45: 10: 45) for 15- 30 mint.
5. The precipitation lines or band will take dark blue colour.

Interpretations

Three basic pattern of results are observed in AGPT

Reaction of identity: it occurs between identical antigenic determinants. The lines of precipitation fuse to form one continuous line in the area.

Reaction of non-identity: Two lines are formed independently without any interaction when two antigens do not contain any common antigenic determinant.

Reaction of partial identity: Spur is formed when some of the determinants are common.

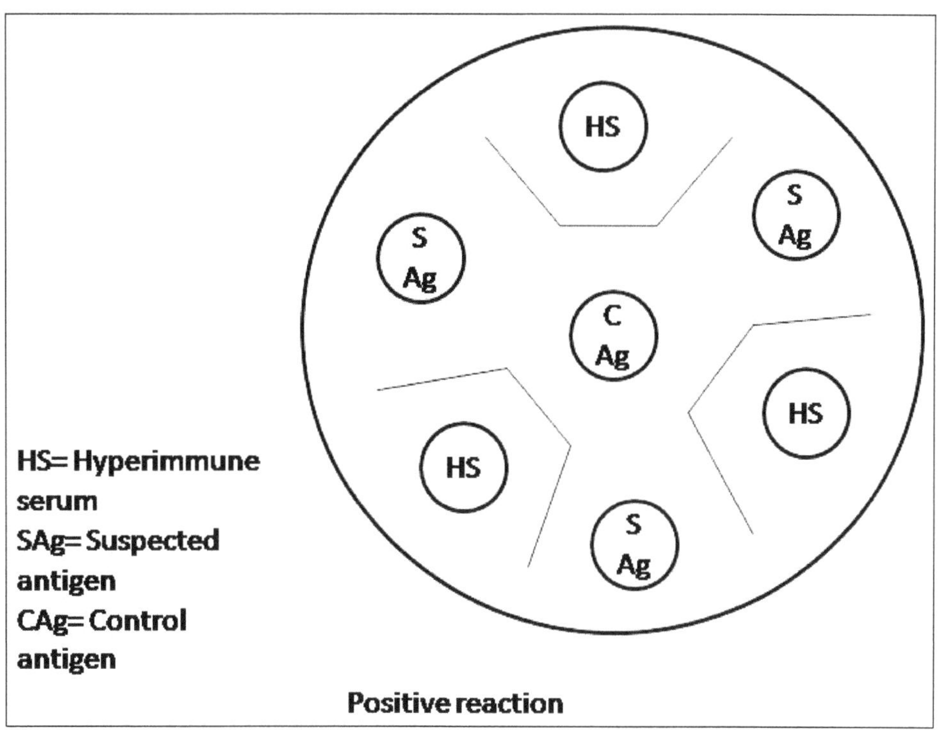
HS
S
Ag
S
Ag
C
Ag
HS
HS
S
Ag
HS= Hyperimmune
serum
SAg= Suspected
antigen
CAg= Control
antigen
Positive reaction

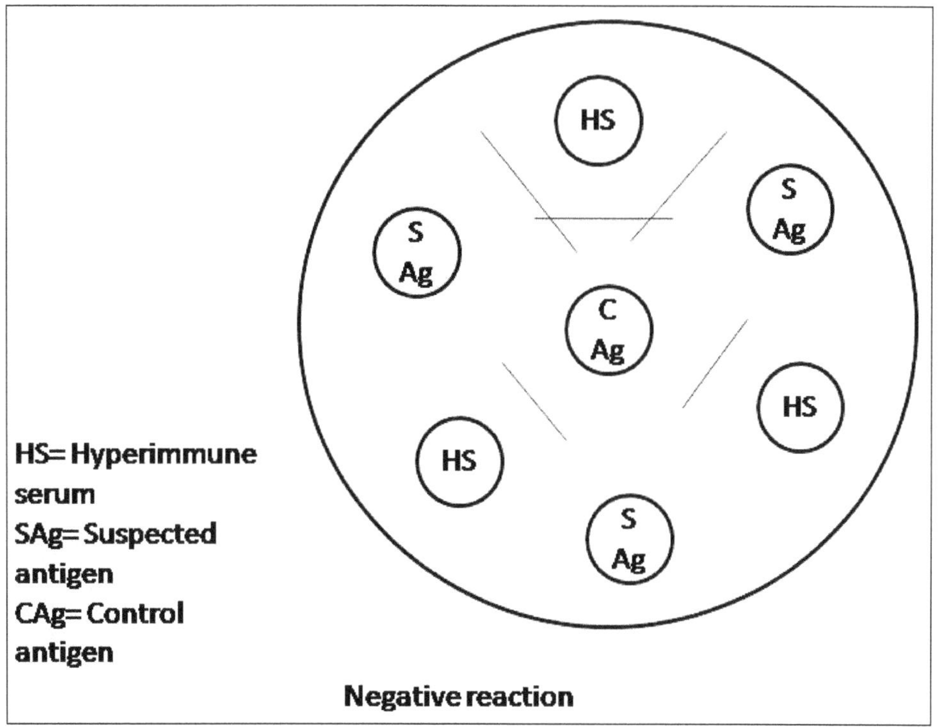
HS
S
Ag
S
Ag
C
Ag
HS
HS
S
Ag
HS= Hyperimmune
serum
SAg= Suspected
antigen
CAg= Control
antigen
Negative reaction

Agglutination Tests

It is a type of serological reaction in which antibodies react with particulate antigen and form visible clump. This test is used to detect the presence (qualitative) or to detect amount of unknown antigen in serum sample or specific antigen.

Types

1. Tube Agglutination Test or TAT
2. Slide Agglutination Test or SAT.

Tube Agglutination Test (TAT)

It is quantitative test which is employed to determine the titer of antibodies in an unknown serum sample. Constant amount of antigen is mixed with various dilutions of antibodies to show visible clump. Titer is recorded as the highest dilution of serum giving visible reaction.

Materials

Bacterial antigen, Specific agglutination serum, NSS, Serological tubes (agglutination tubes/Dryer's tube), Graduated pipettes (1 ml) 10 in number.

Procedure

1. Arrange 11 serological tubes in a rack and mark them 1 to 11 (10 for test and 11th as control).
2. Add 0.9 ml of NSS in 1st tube and 0.5 ml of NSS in tube no. 2 to 11.
3. Add 0.1 ml of serum in 1st tube, mix well and take 0.5 ml of the contents and add to 2nd tube.
4. Repeat the process up to tube no. 10 and discard 0.5 ml of the contents from tube no 10. Leave the tube no. 11 undisturbed (without serum dilution), as shown in the table.
5. Add 0.5 ml of antigen solution to each tube.
6. Mix well the each tube and incubate at 37°C for 24 hours.

Tubes	*1*	*2*	*3*	*4*	*5*	*6*	*7*	*8*	*9*	*10*	*11 (control)*
Saline	0.9	0.5	0.5	0.5	0.5	0.5	0.5	0.5	0.5	0.5	0.5
Serum	0.1	0.5 →	0.5 →	0.5 →	0.5 →	0.5 →	0.5 →	0.5 →	0.5 →	0.5 →	****
	Mix saline and serum in the sample in tube one and transfer 0.5 ml of solution in tube no. 2 mix and repeat the process for tube no 3 to 10 serially discard 0.5 ml from tube no 10										
Antigen	0.5	0.5	0.5	0.5	0.5	0.5	0.5	0.5	0.5	0.5	0.5
Final contents	1.0 ml	1.0 ml	1.0 ml	1.0 ml	1.0 ml	1.0 ml	1.0 ml	1.0 ml	1.0 ml	1.0 ml	1.0 ml
Dilution	1:10	1:20	1:40	1:80	1:160	1:320	1:640	1:1280	1:2560	1:5120	****

Results

Agglutination reaction is recorded as the presence of sediment (clump) in tube. Control tube is examined for uniform turbidity and ensures the absence of any agglutinate.

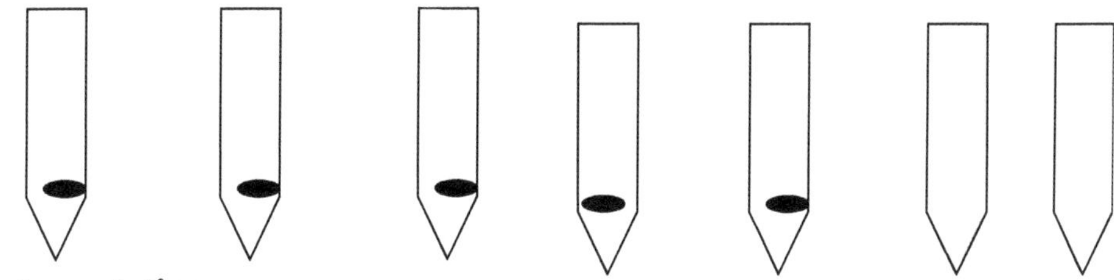

Interpretation

- ☆ Degree of agglutination is judged by the opacity of fluid. Higher the agglutination less the opacity.
- ☆ The highest dilution of serum which produces the agglutination of antigen is considered as the end point.

Plate/Slide Agglutination Test (SAT)

It is qualitative test which is employed to detect the presence of an unknown antibody in a serum sample or unknown antigen in a solution. This test is mainly useful in screening bacterial and viral diseases in a flock or herd but it is not suitable for specific identifications.

Principle

When particulate antigen is mixed with antibodies in the presence of electrolyte at suitable temperature and pH the particulate antigen clumps and form agglutination. Size of particle should have more than 25 nm to produce a visible reaction.

Materials

Glass plate, Stirring rod coloured antigen, Suspected serum samples, Positive serum negative serum.

Procedure

1. Place one drop of unknown antiserum and one drop of known antigen side by side on an agglutination plate.
2. Mix the drop with a matchstick and rotate the plate by tilting the sides.
3. Agglutination reaction is noted by formation of clumps in the solution
4. Control antigen is mixed with NSS to check for auto agglutination.

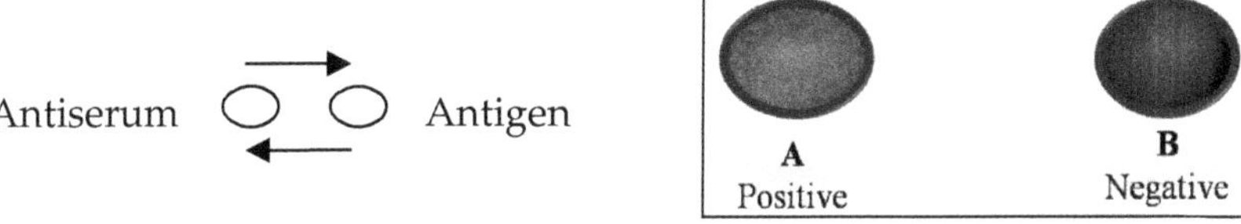

Interpretation

Presence of agglutination shows the presence of specific antibodies in the unknown serum.

Advantages

1. It is simpler to perform and easily visible than the precipitation test.
2. It is a rapid and convenient method for determining the presence of agglutinating antibodies and preliminary used for screening of diseases like salmonellosis, brucellosis and mycoplasma infection in a flock or herd.

Disadvantage

1. It is qualitative test, can't measure the quantity of antibodies.
2. It is not suitable when the mixture of organisms and antibodies are present in the sample.

Applications

- ☆ Diagnosis of various bacterial, viral diseases.
- ☆ Identification and typing of bacterial isolates.

Haemagglutination (HA) Test

> The test does not discriminate between viral particles that are infectious and particles that are degraded and no longer able to infect cells.

Principle

Some virus particles have an envelope protein called the hemagglutinin, or HA, which binds to receptors on the membrane of red blood cells. The linking together of the red blood cells by the viral particles results in clumping. This clumping is known as haemagglutination. Haemagglutination is visible macroscopically and is the basis of haemagglutination tests to detect the presence of viral particles.

> Haemagglutination positive virus
> Orthomyxoviruses,
> Paramyxoviruses,
> Togaviruses (including rubella),
> Flaviviruses,
> Bunyaviruses.

Materials

Micro Titer plate V bottom

Saline

Micro pipette

Micro Tips

1 per cent chicken RBC

Alserver's Solution

Preperation of Alserver's Solution

Dextrose	2.05g
Sodium Chloride	0.420g
Sodium Citrate	0.800g

Citric acid 0.055g

Distilled Water 100ml.

Mix properly and sterilize in syringe filter and store at 40°C..

Preparation of Washed Chick R.B.C. (1 per cent)

1. Take 9 ml of Alserver's solution and add 1ml of blood from chick (up to 3-4 days) in a test tube.
2. Then put the test tube on one hole of the centrifuge and in opposite direction, taken same amount of normal saline (0.9 per cent NaCl).
3. Centrifuge 1500 r.p.m for 10 minutes.
4. Discard the upper portion of clotted part and add same amount of normal saline and centrifuge as before.
5. In this way, wash blood 4-5 times.
6. Take 1ml R.B.C pellets and add 99ml of normal saline *i.e.* 1 per cent washed chick R.B.C.

H.A Test Procedure

1. Take a 'V' bottom shaped 96 well plates.
2. Add 50µl normal saline (0.9 per cent Nacl) in each well of the first row and second row.
3. Take Lasoto virus strain or isolated strain and add 4ml of normal saline.
4. Then add 50µl of the virus in first well and serial dilution is done and discard 50µl from 12th well.
5. Then add 50µl of 1 per cent washed chick R.B.C. to each well first row and second row.
6. Then wait for mat and button formation.

Interpretations

+ ve case – matt formation

2nd row button formation (as it is control)

In 1st row button formation in few wells (last)

Antigen titre: inverse of highest dilution of virus dilution which form matt(heamagglutinate the RBC)

Calculations

If matt disappear after the 6th well than

Antigen titer = 64, as after 64 there is button formation.

Calculation of 8 HA virus = 64/8 =8

Then 7ml of normal saline (0.9 per cent NaCl) and 1ml of virus is mixed and we get 8HA virus.

Haemagglutination Inhibition (HI) Test

The basis of the haemagglutination Inhibition assay is that presence of antibodies to that particular virus (for example-influenza virus) will prevent attachment (haemagglutination) of the virus to RBC.

Procedure

1. Add 25µl normal saline (0.9 per cent NaCl) to each well of the row.
2. Add 25µl serum in 1st well of the row and make serial dilution.
3. Add 25µl 4HA virus to each well of the row.
4. Incubate the plate at room temperature for 30 minutes.
5. Then add 25µl 1 per cent washed chick R.B.C to each well.

Interpretations

Positive reaction: Button formation

Negative reaction: Matt formation

Calculations

Antibodies titre

If button formation up to 5tubes then Ab titer =2x16 =32

ELISA (Enzyme Linked Immuno Sorbent Assay)

Enzyme linked immuno sorbent assay (ELISA) is an analytical method, designed to combine the specificity of antibodies with the sensitivity of simple enzyme assays, by using antibodies to detect the presence of an antibody or an antigen in a wet or liquid sample. ELISAs are designed for detection and quantitative estimation of substance such as peptides, proteins, antibodies, hormones, haptens, drugs and their metabolites. ELISAs can provide a useful measurement of antigen or antibody concentration.

There are two main variations on this method:

1. The ELISA to detect the presence of antigens that are recognized by an antibody or
2. The ELISA to test for antibodies that recognize an antigen.

Advantages of ELISA

1. Easy to perform once trained in the procedure.
2. Small quantity of reagent required which can process large number of sample at a time.
3. Can be modified and standardized according to the test and purpose.
4. Result produce in the form of coloured reaction which can easily read by naked eye and result can also be easily quantified by spectrophotometers.
5. It is quite sensitivity (0.01 to 1 µg/ml) and specific test.

6. Reagents used in this procedure are readily available, safe and non mutagenic.
7. It can be performed at anywhere, even in laboratories where facilities are very low.

Materials

ELISA Plate: 96 well flat bottomed wells microtitre plate made up of polyvinyl chloride or polystyrene is commonly used.

Antigen, test serum

Conjugate: Horse radish peroxidase (HRP), Alkaline phosphatase (AP), Beta galactosidase Urease anti-immunoglobulin conjugate.

Chromogen Substrate: It imparts coloure in presence of enzyme conjugate. The rate of colour development will be proportional to the amount of enzyme conjugate present.

Enzyme	*Substrate*	*Chromogen*	*Buffer*	*Stopping Agent*	*Colour*
Horse Radish-peroxidase (HRP)	Hydrogen peroxide (H_2O_2) (0.004%)	Orthophenylene diamine dihydrochloride (OPD)	Phosphate/ Citrate, pH 5.0	1M H_2SO_4	Orange/ Brown
Alkaline Phosphatase (AP)	Paranitrophenyl phosphate (PNP)	Paranitrophenyl phosphate (PNP)	Diethanola-mine, pH 9.8	3M NaOH	Yellow/ green

Coating Buffer

Bicarbonate/Carbonate (100 mM)

3.03 g Na_2CO_3

6.0 g $NaHCO_3$

1000 ml distilled water,

pH 9.6

Blocking Solution

1 per cent BSA or Serum or 5 per cent skimmed milk power or casein or gelatin in PBS.

Wash Solution

PBS or Tris -buffered saline (pH 7.4) with detergent such as 0.05 per cent (v/v) Tween20

Phosphate Buffer Saline (PBS)

pH 7.4

1.16 g Na_2HPO_4

0.1 g KCl

0.1 g K_3PO_4

4.0 g NaCl (500 ml distilled water)

Stopping Agent

1M H_2SO_4 or 3M NaOH commonly used stopping agent to stop the coloure development reaction.

ELISA Reader

Antibody dilution buffer: Primary and secondary antibody should be diluted in 1x blocking solution to reduce non-specific binding.

Five Basic Steps in ELISA Procedure

1. Coating of micro titer plate wells with antigen
2. Blocking of unbound sites to prevent false positive results
3. Addition of primary antibody (Rabbit monoclonal antibody) in wells
4. Addition of secondary antibody conjugated to an enzyme
5. Reaction of a substrate with the enzyme to produce a colored product, for positive reaction

Types of ELISA

1. Direct ELISA
2. Indirect ELISA
3. Sandwich ELISA
4. Competitive ELISA
5. Multiplex ELISA

Direct ELISA Procedure

1. Coat ELISA plate wells with testing antigen

   Note: Preparation of testing antigen (10 µg/ml to 0.01 ng/ml in 50 mM Na_2C0_3, pH 9.6, adjust based on the reactivity of antibody).
2. Incubate the plate after sealing for overnight at 4 C.
3. Wash plate 3 times with PBS-T (0.05 per cent Tween-20 in PBS).
4. Block plate with 0.2 per cent non-fat dry milk in PBS at room temperature for 1 hour at 4 C
5. Wash plate 3 times with PBS-T.
6. Incubate with biotinylated, affinity-purified rabbit IgG (0.1-0.5 µg/ml in PBS, 100 µl/well) at room temperature for 1 hour, followed by washing 6 times with PBS-T.
7. Incubate with HRP-Streptavidin (1:4000-10,000 dilutions) in 0.2 per cent milk-PBS, 100 µl/well, at room temperature for 1 hour.

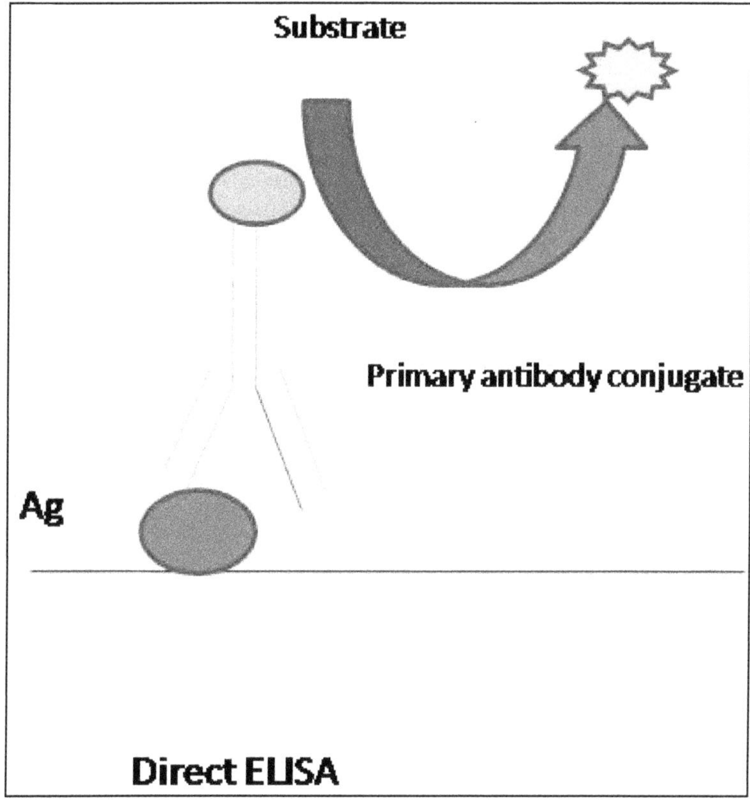

8. Wash plate 8 times with PBS-T.
9. Develop color using TMB as a substrate (100 µl/well) and incubate at room temperature for 15-30 minutes without shaking.
10. Stop reaction by addition of 2N H_2S0_4 (100 µl/well). Record the absorbance at 450 nm on a plate reader within 30 minutes of stopping the reaction.

Indirect ELISA

The Indirect-ELISA utilizes both primary and secondary antibody. Primary antibody is unlabeled which bind to coated antigen. The labeled secondary antibody is directed against all antibodies of a given species, it can be used with a wide variety of primary antibodies.

Step

Coating of Antigen

Fill Wells of ELISA plate with antigen solution (20µl) and incubate at 4°C in a humid chamber over night. (Dissolve antigen in carbonate-bicarbonate buffer (pH 9.4) to obtain antigen concentration of 5-10 µl/ml). This process occurs though hydrophobic interactions between the micro titer plate and non-polar protein residues.

Washing

Wash the wells twice with PBS-Tween (assay buffer). It is necessary to remove nonbound reagents and decrease background insufficient washing lead to high background, while excessive washing might result in decreased sensitivity.

Blocking Buffer

Add 20µl of 1 per cent BSA to each well and incubate at 37°C for 1 hour. Residual binding capacity of the plate is blocked in this step as the binding capacity of microplate wells is typically higher than the amount of protein coated in each well. The blocking buffer improves the sensitivity of an assay by reducing non specific binding of antibodies.

Primary Antibody Addition

Add 200 µl of diluted test serum as well as standard antibody solution (diluted in assay buffer, 2 µl of antibody + 2 µl of assay buffer) and incubate for 2 hours at 37°C in a humid environment and. The antibody is usually diluted in blocking buffer to prevent non specific attachment of protein in the antiserum on the solid phase.

Washing

Excess antibody or unbound antibodies are removed by washing the wells thrice with assay buffer step.

Secondary Antibody (Antibody Enzyme Conjugate) Addition

Add 200 µl of diluted per oxidase immunoglobulin conjugate (Secondary antibody) directed against the primary antibody to each well.

Washing

Wash the wells thrice with assay buffer.

Substrates Adding

Add 200 µl of substrate solution to each well and allow acting for 15-30 minutes at room temperature in dark. The objective is to allow development of coloure reaction through enzyme catalysis. Many substrates are available for performing the ELISA with an HRP or AP conjugate. The choice depends upon sensitivity needed for the that assay and the instrumentation available (spectrophotometer, fluorometer).

Stopping the Reaction

Add 50 µl of 5N NaOH solution (for AP conjugate) or 0.2 M sulphuric acid (for HRPO conjugate) for to each well to stop the reaction. Stop Solution is a used to terminate the enzyme substrate reaction after attaining the desired color intensity which is an indication of analyte level.

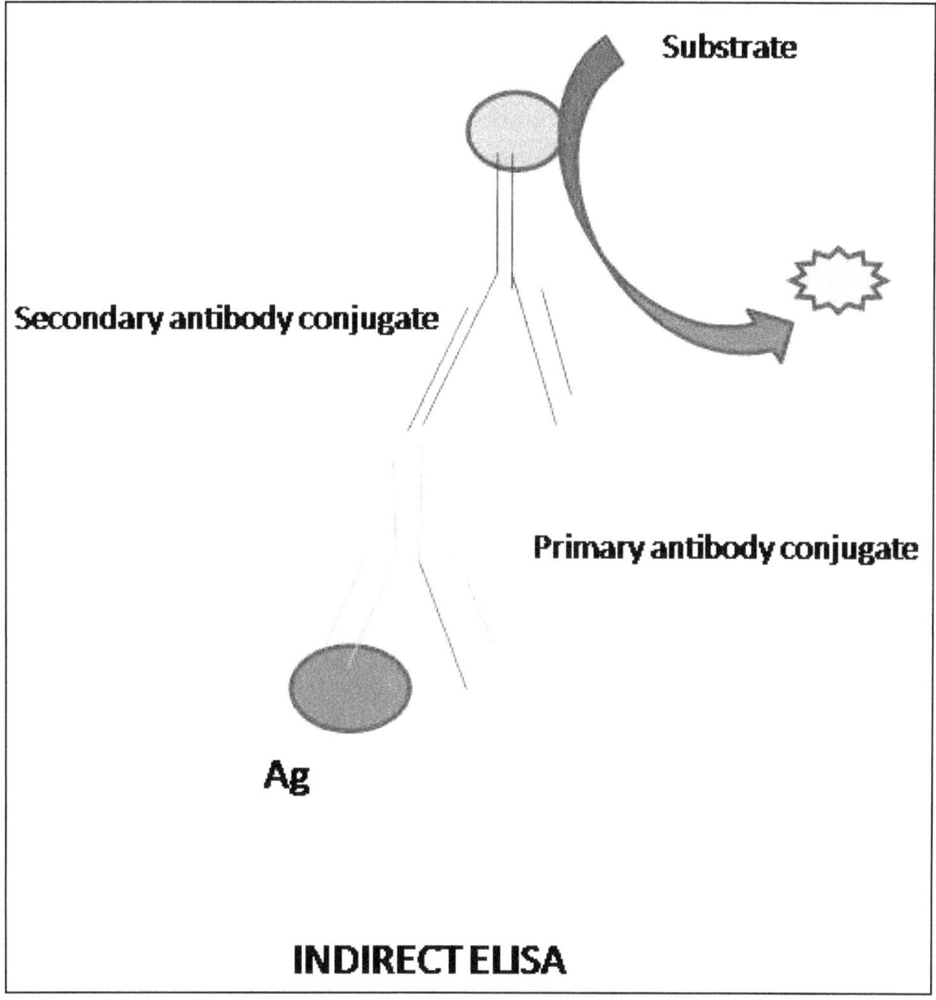

Reading

Record the absorbance at 450 (A 450) nm on a plate reader within 30 minutes of stopping the reaction.

Calculations

Prepare a standard curve of concentration of standard antibody Vs A450 on a graph paper by taking concentration of antibody on X-axis and A450 on Y-axis. Determine the concentration of test sample from the graph.

Advantages

- Indirect ELISA test is highly sensitivity in this more than one labeled antibody is bound per antigen molecule.
- Fewer labeled antibodies are required so it is cost saving test.

Competitive ELISA

Competitive ELISA is another method of ELISA that involves competitive bidding process executed by original antigen (sample antigen) and add-in antigen. Higher the sample antigen concentration, the weaker the eventual signal.

Note: The labeled antigen competes for primary antibody binding sites with sample antigen (unlabeled). The more antigens in the sample the less labeled antigen is retained in the well and the weaker the signal).

Procedure

1. Incubate unlabeled antibody within presence of its antigen.
2. Bound antibody/antigens are added to an antigen coated well.
3. Wash and remove unbound antibodies.
4. Competition results from the fact that the more antigens are present in the sample, the fewer antibodies will be able to bind.
5. A secondary antibody that is coupled to an enzyme is added.
6. Substrate added for signal
7. The weaker colored or fluorescent signal that is released shows that that the original antigen concentration was high.

Advantages

- ☆ Competitive ELISA has ability to use crude or impure samples and still selectively bind any antigen that may be present.
- ☆ Suitable for complex samples, since the antigen does not require purification prior to measurement
- ☆ High specificity, since two antibodies are used the antigen/analyte is specifically captured and detected

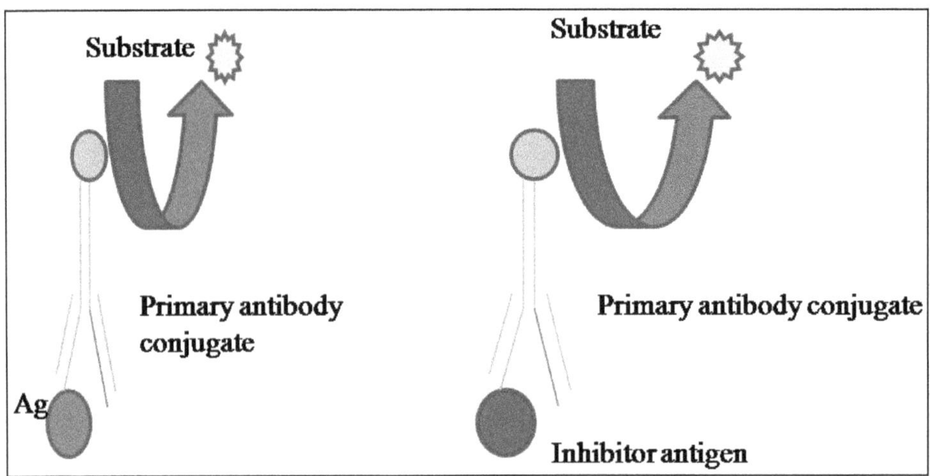

Sandwich ELISA

Principle

In the Sandwich ELISA, or two site capture assay, two different antibodies are used. The wells are coated with an antibody specific for one region of the antigen, then the test solution containing antigen is added. Following washing, the second antibody, which recognizes a different epitope of the antigen, will be added. This antibody will have the enzyme attach.

Procedure

Before the assay, both antibody preparations should be purified and one must be labeled. For most applications, a polyvinylchloride (PVC) micro titer plate is best.

- Coat the ELISA plate with diluted capture antibody and incubate overnight at 4 C.
- Wash the plate wells with PBS-Triton twice.
- Block non-specific binding using 1 per cent BSA/PBS and incubate for 30-60 minutes at RT.
- Wash the plate and add standards and 100ul of diluted samples to appropriate wells.
- Incubate for 1 hour at RT and wash wells.
- Add 100ul appropriate dilution of the secondary antibody conjugated with Alkaline Phosphatase (AP) or Horseradish Peroxidase (HRP) and incubate for 1 hour and wash wells.
- Add 100ul of substrate to well and incubate at RT for 1 hour. (Add stopping solution)
- Read plates on an ELISA micro plate reader.

Advantages

- High specificity, since two antibodies are used the antigen/analyte is specifically captured and detected
- Suitable for complex samples, since the antigen does not require purification prior to measurement
- Flexibility and sensitivity, since both direct and indirect detection methods can be used
- Sandwich ELISA is a common tool to diagnose Influenza, e.g. H5N1 (Avian Flu) Hemagglutinin ELISA kit.
- In addition, a description of the application of sandwich ELISA to home pregnancy test can be found here.

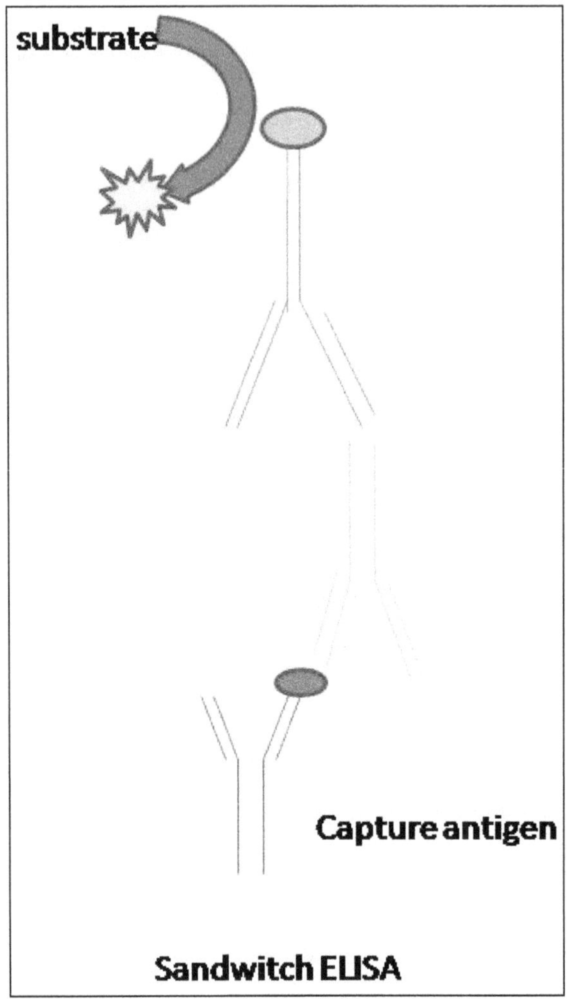

Dot Immuno Assay

Dot Immuno Assay is a technique for detecting, analyzing, and identifying proteins spotted through circular templates directly onto the membrane. It is similar to the western blot technique but differing in that protein samples are not separated electrophoretically.

Principle

Proteins (antigen) are onto a (nitrocellulose membrane or nylon). The antigen is immobilized solid support by dotting into the nitrocellulose membrane and then incubated with test antibody and subsequently with secondary antibody conjugated with enzyme. Bounds conjugate gives colour when treated with substrate.

Materials

Nitrocellulose membrane (NCM), Anti-immunoglobulins conjugated with Horse Radish Peroxidase enzyme, Diamino benzidine (DAB) -Prepared by mixing 10 mg of DAB with 50 ml of Tris buffer and adding 20 µl of 30 per cent hydrogen peroxide, Phosphate buffered saline, pH 7.2 (PBS), Micropipettes, Sample for antigen, Dried milk powder, Phosphate buffered saline with Tween (0.1 per cent) (PBST), Serum (Positive and negative control).

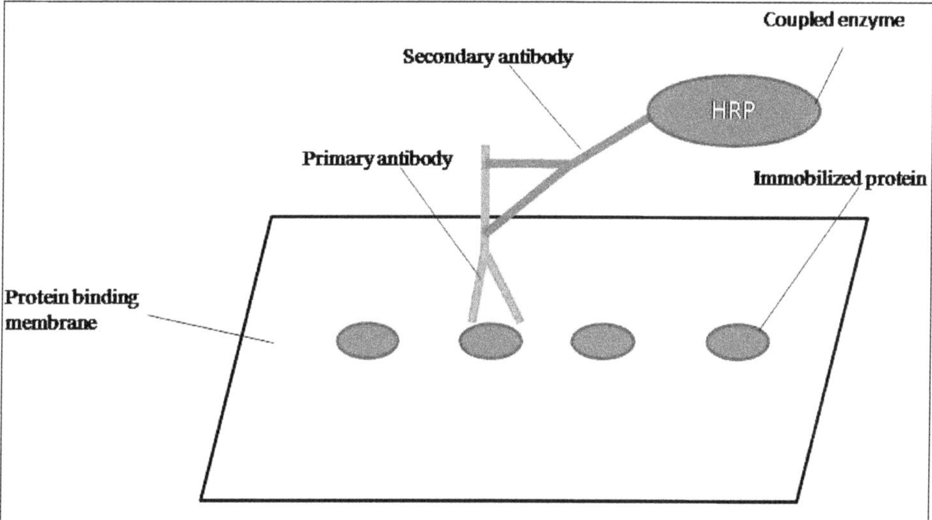

Procedure

Preparation of Nitrocellulose Membrane (Solid Phase Matrix)

Take nitrocellulose membrane (0.22µm or 0.45 µm pore size) ready, draw grid by pencil to indicate the region you are going to blot

Dotting of Antigen

1. Using micropipette spot 2 µl of samples onto the nitrocellulose membrane at the center of the grid.
2. Let the membrane air dried.

Blocking

Block non-specific sites by soaking in 5 per cent BSA in TBS-T or 5 per cent dried milk powder in PBST and incubated at 37°C for 1 hr.

Serum Sample

Incubate with primary antibody (1:100 to 1:1000 dilution for antisera in BSA/ TBS-T for 1 hr at 37°C and wash three times with TBS-T (3 x 5 min).

Conjugate

- Incubate with secondary antibody conjugated with HRP (for optimum dilution, follow the manufacturer's recommendation) for 1 hr at 37°C.
- Wash three times with TBS-T (15 min x 1, 5 min x 2), then once with TBS (5 min).

Substrate Solution

- Incubate the membrane in substrate solution of DAB, until spots are visible.
- Stop the reaction – rinse the membrane in distilled water. Air dries the membrane.

Interpretations

In positive cases, a brown spot appears at the site of application of sample, the intensity of the color is proportional to the concentration of the antigen.

Advantage

- Procedure is simple and no special instruments are required for reading. The development of colored dot at the site can be visualized with naked eyes
- Nitrocellulose membrane dotted with antigen can be stored for a few months at 4-8°C.

Applications

- Identification and characterizations of protein.
- Identification of infectious agents present in the sample.

Chapter 17

Isolation and Identification of Mycotic Pathogens

Fungi, yeasts and moulds are widespread throughout the environment. Animal get affected to these agents in poor unhygienic conditions, stress, prolong antibiotic treatment and immunosuppressive infection. Mycotic infection can be cutaneous, subcutaneous and even systemic. Sometime laboratory diagnosis by isolation and identification of fungal species is very important to differentiate it from some bacterial infection and to determine the proper treatment regime.

Isolation Methods

Culture on Media

Principles

Fungi are generally classified into molds and yeast. Moulds are multicellular, filamentous and produce spores on brightly colored aerial hyphae while yeasts are unicellular in nature and produces bacterial like colony on media. Fungi grow at comparatively slow rates, often requiring several days to weeks to form macroscopically visible colonies on media. Most molds grow best at room temperature (25 C) and pH 5.6 rather than at 37 C. Sabouraud dextrose agar is basic media generally used for culturing many mold. Presence of high sugar concentration and low pH (5.6) prevent the growth of most bacteria and contaminate. Fungi are identified primarily by examining their reproductive structures, morphological characteristics, and colony growth.

Media

Sabouraud Dextrose Agar (pH-5.6)

Peptone	10g
Dextrose	40g
Agar	15g
Distilled water	1lit

Procedure

1. Melt Sabouraud dextrose agar powder in distilled water.
2. Cool to 48 to 50 C in a water bath.
3. Pour into petri plates and allow hardening.
4. Using aseptic technique, inoculate the plates with collected clinical sample without spreading it.
5. Incubate the plate at room temperature for 2 to 5 days. Do not invert the petri plates.
6. Each day examine the plate for growth.
7. If colony appears on the plate then perform microscopic examinations for the identifications.

Slide Culture Technique

Principle

Wet mount slides made from mold colonies usually don't reveal the arrangement of spores that is so necessary in identification. Also in the process of merely transferring hyphae to a slide breaks the hyphen and sporangiophores. In slide cultures fungi directly grow on the slide on a thin film of agar. So, there is no need to remove a portion of the fungus from a culture plate and transfer it to the slide. Slide culture technique provide better option to identify the fungus characteristic as hyphae, sporangiophores, and spores remain more or less intact when stained.

Materials

Sterile Petri dish, Filter paper, U-shaped glass rod, Microscope slides and coverslips (Sterile), SDA plate, Lactophenol cotton blue stain, Scalpel, Inoculating needle, Sterile distilled water, 95 per cent ethanol, Forceps.

Procedure

1. Do all the procedure aseptically.
2. Place a sheet of sterile filter paper in a Petri dish with the help of forceps.
3. Place a sterile U-shaped glass rod on the filter paper.
4. Pour sterile water on the filter paper to completely moisten it.
5. Place a sterile slide on the U-shaped rod with the help of forceps.
6. Cut a 5 mm square block of the SDA medium by the sterilize scalpel.
7. Transfer this block aseptically to the centre of the slide.
8. Pick up spores or mycelial fragments of the fungus to be examined and inoculate on the four sides of the agar square.
9. Place a sterile cover glass on the agar cube.
10. Cover the Petri dish and incubate at room temperature for 48-72 hours.
11. After 48 hours, examine the slide under microscope as such or after staining with lactophenol cotton blue.

12. For staining add a drop of 95 per cent ethanol to the hyphae on the cover glass.
13. Place a drop of LCB stain on glass slide.
14. As soon as most of the alcohol has evaporated place the cover glass, mold side down, on the drop of lactophenol cotton blue stain on the slide.
15. Examine the slide under microscope.

Interpretations

Characteristic	*Suspected Fungi*
Septate hypae branching at 45° angles	*Aspergillus* spp.
Hypae devoid of septa	Mucor-rhizopus
Small and regular hypae, some branching with rectangular arthrospores sometimes seen, isolated from skin, nail scrapings and hair lesions	*Dermatophyte* spp.
Budding yeast forms (blastospores) and pseudohyphae found	*Candida* spp.
Yeast forms, cell spherical and irregular in size, encapsualted with thick polysaccharide capsule with one or more buds attached by a narrow constriction	*Cryptococcus neoformans*
Small budding yeast with a single bud attached by a narrow base	*Histoplasma capsulatum*
Yeast forms, double contoured wall, with a single bud attached by a broad base	*Blastomyces dermatitidis*
Large, thick walled spherules, containing small round endospores	*Coccidiodes immitis*

Identification

Lacto Phenol Cotton Blue Staining

Principle

Lactophenol cotton blue stain use for staining the fungi in which phenol act as is fungicidal, Lactic acid acts as a preservative which preserves the structure of fungus element and cotton blue act as a staining agent which stains the fungus cytoplasm in light blue colour.

> Mayer's mucicarmine staining is useful technique to identify *Cryptococcus neoformans* and other fungi in tissue sample.

Procedure

1. Add a drop of lactophenol cotton blue solution on a clean grease free slide.
2. Transfer a mycellial mat on fluid with the help of sterilize needle and mix with the stain.
3. Place the cover slip on mycellial mat.
4. Take a blotting paper and wipe the excess stain.
5. Observe under low to high power objectives of microscope.

Periodic Acid Schiff Staining (PAS)

This method is used for detection of fungal infection in tissues. Glycogen, mucin, and fungi will be stained purple and the nuclei will be stained blue with PAS stain.

Procedure

1. Remove paraffin from tissue section and hydrate with water.
2. Oxidize by keeping it in 0.5 per cent periodic acid solution for 5 minutes.
3. Rinse in distilled water.
4. Place in Schiff reagent for 15 minutes.
5. Wash in lukewarm tap water for 5 minutes.
6. Counter stain in Mayer's haematoxylin for 1 minute.
7. Wash in tap water for 5 minutes.
8. Dehydrate and examine under microscope.

Results

Fungi	Red/purple
Background	Blue

Wood's Lamp Method

In this method the affected hairs are viewed directly by UV rays. In Wood's lamp, the light from mercury vapours lamp is filtered through sodium-barium-silicate glass containing nickel oxide. Fluroscence is because of tryptophan metabolits produce by fungus *e.g Microsporum canis.*

Biochemical Reactions

Various type of biochemical test has been utilized for identification of fungus depending of their biochemical properties.

Carbohydrate Fermentation

Specimen is inoculated in the broth and layered with paraffin over top. Bromcresol purple is the indicator. Observe every 48 hours for 14 days..Growth and utilization of a carbohydrate under anaerobic conditions determined by acid and gas production Acid production turns purple to yellow. Gas is detected by appearance of bubbles trapped in the fermentation tube.

Nitrogen Assimilation

Utilizes 3 tubes with differing sources of nitrogen. Bromthymol blue is the indicator (blue to yellow is positive).

Growth on Specific Agars

Christensen's urea agar - Urea is hydrolyzed by some yeast to form ammonia (pH increases) which turns media from yellow to dark pink.

Germ Tube Test

Principle

Candida albicans produce germ tubes within 2 hours in contact with the serum. The germ tube test is used for presumptive identification of *Candida albicans.*

Procedure

> ***Cryptococcus neoformans*** form thick capsule around yeast cell which can be demonstrated by India ink staining.

1. Take a fresh grown pure culture of test oraganism.
2. Make a very light suspension of the test organism in 0.5 ml of sterile serum
3. Incubate at 37 C for exactly 2 hours.
4. Put 1 drop from the incubated serum on a slide with a coverslip.
5. Observe under the microscope for germ tube productions.

Observations

Germ tube: Hyphal growth, arising directly from the yeast cell wall without constriction at origin point.

Chapter 18

Practice for Separation of Toxic Materials from Samples and their Detection from Body Fluids and Tissue of Animals

Most of the toxicosis conditions are acute in nature and lethal to animal. There symptom in animal are mostly generalized in nature. It is very important to investigations toxic condition not only for accurate diagnosis and proper medication but also to solve the veterolegal cases. Increasing trends in use of chemicals in various agriculture and animal husbandry practices increase the possibilities of toxicosis in animals. Commonly sources of poisoning in animals are pesticides, insecticides, herbicides, fertilizers, toxic plants/herbs, industrial effluents, heavy metals and toxic minerals, drugs, chemicals and mycotoxins. Clinically toxicosis occurs after some time when these chemicals are accumulated in tissue of animals. Most of the toxicosis cases are being diagnosed based on the laboratory analysis of clinical sample.

General Point to be Considered while Collecting and Handling Samples for Toxicological Examinations

- ☆ Tissue and suspected material both should be sent to laboratory in sufficient amount.
- ☆ Only one type of material should be kept in sterilized container.
- ☆ Samples should be refrigerated immediately after collection.
- ☆ Transport the material on frozen cool packs only.
- ☆ Normally, preservative is not added to the toxicological material. Most preferred preservative is 95 per cent ethanol@ 1.0 ml/g of sample. The denatured alcohol or formalin should never be used.
- ☆ The sample should be properly labeled with indication of, species of animal/plant, tissue, date and time of death, and preservative added with a written document of all details related with case.

Route of Exposure

1. Inhalation (breathing it into the lungs)
2. Skin contact
3. Ingestion

Specimens Collected for Toxicological Examination

Suspected Poisons	Material Required (Arranged in Order of Significance)
Aflatoxin Mycotoxins	Suspected feed, piece of liver, spleen and kidney in 10 per cent formalin and or ice separately
Ammonia	Whole blood (without ammonium oxalate as anticoagulant) covered with a 1" layer mineral oil. (Test within 12 hours).
Arsenic (acute)	Liver, kidney, stomach and contents of rumen and abomassum and suspected feed.
Arsenic (chronic)	Hair, urine and liver
Carbon tetrachloride	Stomach contents and parenchymatous viscera
Cyanides/ Hydrocyanic acid	Stomach and rumen contents, liver, oxalates or heparinized blood and forage.
Copper	Liver, kidney, feed and whole blood
Fertilizer	Stomach contents and whole blood
Lead	Kidney, liver, blood and stomach contents; bone in chronic cases
Mercury	Kidney, liver and stomach contents
Mineral acid and alkali	Stomach and its contents, liver, kidney and urine
Nitrate and nitrite	Serum, feed and water
Oxalate	Serum, blood and kidney
Phenothiazines	Urine and serum
Pesticides	Body fat and whole blood
Phenol	Stomach and rumen content
Phosphorus	Stomach and rumen content and serum
Selenium	Liver, kidney, hair and hoof
Sodium chloride	serum and Stomach content
Sodium nitrate	Stomach contents and oxalated blood
Strychnine	Stomach contents, liver and urine
Urea	Oxalated whole blood under mineral oil and feed
Warferin	Liver

Quantities of different Materials Required for Toxicological Examination

Specimen	Quantity Required
Blood	10-30 ml
Bone	250 gram
Feed, grain and seeds	500 gram
Fodder	500 gram

Specimen	*Quantity Required*
Feed ingredients	500 gram
Hair	5.0 gram
Kidney	50-200 gram
Liver and spleen	50-200 gram
Serum	5.0 ml
Stomach or rumen contents	100-500 gram

Common Methods Used in Toxicant Extraction

Methods	*Uses*
Blending	Used to separate samples from cell and sub cellular organelles with the help of electrically operated blender and sonicator respectively.
Solid extraction	Separation process, compounds dissolved or suspended in a liquid mixture is separated from other compounds in the mixture according to their physical and chemical properties.
Washing and shaking	Releases contaminants from the surface of solvent.
Continuous Extraction	Used for an exhaustive extraction of the toxicants from the sample.
Liquid -liquid extraction	Solvent extraction method, separate compounds based on their relative solubility in two different immiscible liquids.
Cold extraction	Substance is extracted from a mixture via cold water.
Homogenization	Obtain a suspension or emulsion to form a constant different insoluble phase by blending of mutually related substances.

Various Methods Used in Evaluation and Estimation of Toxic Residues in the Samples

Methods	*Uses*
Gas Chromatography	For the separation of volatile components of mixtures through a column containing a liquid or solid stationary phase by differential migration.
High-Performance Liquid Chromatography	For the separation of components of mixtures through a column containing a micro particulate solid stationary phase by differential migration.
Atomic Absorption Spectrometry	Used widely for the quantitative determination of metals at trace levels with the principle of absorption of electromagnetic radiation by atoms.
Ultra Violet and Visible Spectrum Spectrophotometry	Provides useful analytical information for both inorganic and organic samples with the principle absorption of the electromagnetic spectrum in the ultraviolet and visible regions corresponds to transitions between electronic energy levels

Some of Common Poisoning in Animals and its Antidotes

Poison/Chemical/Drug/Toxin	*Antidote Treatment*
Lead	BAL (British Antilewisite or dimercaprol), calcium disodium EDTA
Mercury	BAL
Arsenic	BAL (dimercaprol), d-penicillamine

Poison/Chemical/Drug/Toxin	*Antidote Treatment*
Iron	Deferoxamine
Zinc	calcium disodium EDTA
Cyanide	Sodium nitrite, sodium thiosulfate
Nitrite, nitrate, chlorate	Methylene blue
Opiates	Nalorphine
Alkaloids	Tannic acids
Fluorides, oxalates	Calcium gluconate
Barbiturate	Bemegride
Copper	Penicillamine molybdenum salts
Molybdenum	Copper
Organophosphate compound	Cholinesterase reactivators (oximes)
Coumarin anticoagulants	Vit K
Ethylene glycol, methyl alcohol	Ethanol

Common Test Procedure to Detect the Poisonous Substances in Samples

Metal	*Procedure*	*Result*
Arsenic	**Test 1:** 1 ml of test solution + a drop of 20 per cent ammonium sulfide	Appearance of yellow fumes slowly
	Test 2: 1 ml of test solution + a drop of 15 per cent potassium iodide solution	No reaction
Lead	**Test 1:** 1 ml of test solution + a drop of 10 per cent ammonium carbonate	Appearance of white colour/precipitate.
	Test 2: 1 ml of test solution + a drop of 20 per cent ammonium sulfide	Appearance of black colour.
	Test 3: 1 ml of test solution + a drop of 15 per cent potassium iodide solution	Appearance of bright yellow colour
Zinc	**Test 1:** 1 ml of test solution + a drop of 10 per cent ammonium carbonate	Appearance of white colour/precipitate
	Test 2: 1 ml of test solution + a drop of 20 per cent ammonium sulfide	Appearance of white colour; soluble in excess
	Test 3: 1ml of test solution + a drop of 15 per cent potassium iodide solution	No reaction
Copper	**Test 1:** 1 ml of test solution + 10 per cent ammonium carbonate solution	Appearance of light blue colour
	Test 2: 1 ml of test solution + 20 per cent ammonium sulfide solution	Appearance of brown colour
Mercury	**Test 1:**1 ml of test solution + 10 per cent ammonium carbonate	Appearance of white colour
	Test 2: 1 ml of test solution + 20 per cent ammonium sulfide	Appearance of black colour

Metal	*Procedure*	*Result*
	Test 3: 1 ml of test solution + 15 per cent potassium iodide solution	Appearance of green colour turning to red colour. In excess, turning to clear solution
Fluorides	Small quantity (1-3 ml) of urine or stomach contents in a test tube + ferric chloride solution (2 per cent) in drops.	Appearance of white turbudity is indicative of fluoride in the sample.
Nitrite in blood	Add 10 ml blood without anticoagulant in 20 ml capacity test tube and place in boiling water bath for 45 minutes. Cool to room temperature and observe the colour	Colour change to Salmon pink
Nitrite in sample	Take sample (1 ml) in a test tube and add concentrated sulphuric acid by the sides of the test tube	Development of brown fumes indicative of nitrite in the sample.
Cyanide	☆ In 100 ml flask take 50 g of finely ground tissue or stomach contents. ☆ Acidify the contents with tartaric acid. ☆ Take a filter paper previously moistened with 10 per cent guaiacol in alcohol and 0.1 per cent of aqueous copper sulfate solution. ☆ Hang the filter paper in the flask so that it does not touch the contents in the flask, plug the mouth of flask and warm gently. ☆ Allow it to stand for 30 minutes. ☆ Observe the colour of the paper	If cyanide is present, blue colour develops

Chapter 19

Appreciation and Differentiation of Symptoms Caused by Various Types of Toxic Materials including Agrochemical Plants and Drugs

Inorganic Poisoning

Inorganic Poisoning	*Major Body System/ Organs Affected*	*Symptoms*
Lead	Nervous system and bone	Acute: Abdominal pain, teeth grinding, staggering gait, rolling eyes, slobbering, muscle spasms, blindness, uncoordinated attempts to climb obstacles, excessive response to external stimuli, head pressing, convulsions, signs of abdominal pain including kicking at the abdomen. Subacute: Dullness, loss of appetite, abdominal pain, diarrhoea.Chronic: Wasting, loss of appetite, anaemia, constipation, recumbency, difficulty breathing.
Copper	Gastrointestine, blood	Acute: Severe gastro-enteritis with colic signs, diarrhoea, haemolysis, haemoglobinuria and rapid dehydration. Chronic: Weak, dull, foetid diarrhoea, jaundice and death after recumbency.
Arsenic	Gastrointestine, Nervous system	Vomiting, restlessness, drooling of saliva, nausea, severe abdominal pain often with bloody diarrhea, muscle weakness, trembling, staggering, severe dehydration, shock, paralysis, coma and death.

Inorganic Poisoning	*Major Body System/ Organs Affected*	*Symptoms*
Selenium	Gastrointestine, nervous system, joint and hoof	Acute: Abnormal movement, dark watery diarrhea, elevated temperature, weak and rapid pulse, labored respiration, bloating and abdominal pain, pale and blue mucous membranes and dilated pupils. Chronic: Water Soluble Selenium: Blind Stagger (wandering, stumbling over objects, anorexia, and visual impairment) Water Insoluble: Alkali Disease (Cracking of hooves, deformed hoof, cracks in tail and horn, lameness, stiffness of joints, loss of hair).
Zinc	Gastrointestine, liver, bone	Pain in gastrointestinal tract, vomition and bloody diarrhoea, abdominal pain, icteric mucous membrane and death. Chronic: Decrease growth rate, fatigue, paresis of hind limb, anaemia and jaundice.
Mercuric	Gastrointestinal, nervous	Stomatitis, pharyngitis, vomition, diarrhoea, dehydration, nervous disturbance, ataxia, incoordination, paresis, blindness followed by shock and death. Surviving animals show oliguria and azotemia. Organo-mercurials show neurologic signs. Abnormal posture and paralysis occurs before death.

Organic Poisoning

Organic Poisoning	*Major Body System/ Organs Affected*	*Symptoms*
Nitrate poisoning	Blood	Cyanosis, weak and rapid pulse, dyspneoa, hypothermia, brownish discoloration of the blood, tremors, weakness, ataxia, recumbency and death.
Organo-phosphate	Whole body	Muscarinic effect: Miosis, nausea, vomiting diarrhoea, salivation, lacrimation, bradycardia, abdominal pain, diaphoresis, urinary incontinence, fecal incontinence. Nicotinic effect: Muscle fasciculation, paralysis, muscle weakness, hypertension, tachycardia. Central nervous effect: Unconsciousness, confusion, toxic psychosis seizures, fatigue, respiratory depression, dysarthria, ataxia.
Urea	Gastrointestinal	Muscle twitching, teeth grinding, frothy salivation, bloat, colic, frequent urination, forced rapid breathing, staggering, bellowing and terminal seizure activity. Often, animals are found dead near the source of the urea supplement
Phosphorus	Gastrointestinal, bone	Acute: Garlic odour breath, vomition, haemorrhagic diarrhoea, colic and hepatic failure lead to convulsions and death. Chronic: Phossy jaw (poor wound healing and beak down of jaw bone). Wound fails to heal and there is an offensive discharge, necrosis in bone lead to sequestrum formation.
Nitrate	Circulatory	Acute: Subnormal body temperature, muscular tremors, ataxia, brown cyanotic coloration of mucous membrane, dyspnoea, frequent urination, collapse, coma and clonic convulsions. Chronic: Poor weight gain, decreased milk production, abortion and still birth.
Sodium chloride	Nervous, excretory	Appear unwell, lack of appetite and reluctant to drink, increased urination followed by urinary incontinence, pruritis, salivation, nasal discharge, or polyuria, diarrhoea, vomition and nervous signs (tremor hyperesthesia, blindness, circling movement, shivering, seizures,incoordination, wobbly in the legs, ataxia, swaying and walking backward, dragging of hind leg and knuckling at the fetlocks). Pig: Dull depress, dog sit position (opisthotonus), nystagmus, sudden death. Poultry: Wet litter, poor weight gain and feed conversion, weakness, ascitis and paralysis.
Fluoride	Teeth and bone	Reduced feed and water intake lameness, enlargement of bones, stiff gait, rough hair coat, anorexia, mottled and chalky teeth uneven surface, deformity in ribs.
Nitrate and Nitrite	Circulatory and nervous	Acute: Subnormal body temperature, muscular tremors, ataxia, brown cyanotic mucous membrane, dyspnoea, frequent urination, collapse, coma and clonic convulsions. Chronic: Poor weight gain, decreased milk production, abortion and still birth.

Insecticide Poisoning

Insecticide Poisoning	*Major Body System/ Organs Affected*	*Symptoms*
Organochlorine	Gastrointestinal, excretory, nervous	Acute: Profuse salivation, vomition, diarrhoea, urination, sweating, dilation of eyelid (mydriasis), eyelids and face twitching which extends to whole body. Uncontrolled movements, stagger, circling movement, head pressing, abnormal postures, opisthotonus position, intermittent clonic-tonic seizures, paddling and clamping and locking of jaws are common in advanced stages. Death may occur due to respiratory failure. Chronic: mostly chronic toxicity occur due to release of organochlorine from fat depots of the body. Symptom same as acute but in mild form
Carbamate	Gastrointestinal, excretory, nervous	Cyanosis of mucous membrane, hypersalivation, lacrimation, urination, diarrhea, abdominal pain, vomiting, diarrhea, dyspnoea, miosis, sweating, muscle tetany followed by weakness and paralysis. Respiratory failure and hypoxia due to broncho constriction lead to death.
Pyrethroids	Nervous, respiratory	Tremors, incoordination, elevated body temperature, increased aggressive behavior, coughing, wheezing, shortness of breath, runny or stuffy nose, chest pain or difficulty breathing on inhalation.
Amitraz	Gastrointestinal, respiratory	Lethargy, ataxia, sedation, bradycardia, hypothermia, mydriasis, tachypnea/dyspnoea, diarrhoea, vomiting, hypersalivation, dehydration, hypoperfusion, disorientation seizures.

Herbicide Toxicity

Herbicide	*Major Body System/ Organs Affected*	*Symptoms*
	Gastrointestinal	Cattle: Rumen stasis, bloat, depression, muscular weakness, lameness in hind limb Dogs and Pigs: Diarrhoea, excessive salivation and periodic spasms
Dinitro compounds/ Dinitrophenols	Respiratory	Acute: Fever, restlessness, dyspnea, loss of appetite, thirst, tachycardia, weakness, prostration, cyanosis, hyperthermia, convulsions, coma and death. Chronic: Cataract, restlessness, excess thirst and loss of weight
Bipyridyls compounds	Gastrointestinal, respiratory	Diquat (mainly GIT affected): Anorexia, gastritis, watery diarrhoea, dehydration, nervous excitement, renal failure convulsions and death occur in severely affected animals. Paraquat (both GIT and lung affected): Initially toxicity causes gastroenteritis after progression cause pulmonary oedema and alveolar fibrosis. Other symptoms are tachycardia, tachypnoea dehydration, respiratory sounds and emphysema.

Rodenticide Poisoning

Rodenticide	*Major Body System/ Organs Affected*	*Symptoms*
Zinc Phosphide	Gastrointestinal, nervous	Bloody vomiting, abdominal pain, depression, tremors, dyspnoea, gasping, struggling, convulsions or hyperesthesia, hyperthermia coma and death Dogs: Aimless running, howling, barking, snapping of teeth, tremors and salivation. Horses: Colic Cattle: Bloat
Sodium Fluoro-acetate and Sodium Fluoro-cetamide	Nervous, cardiac	Dogs (CNS mainly affected): Restlessness, hyperirritability, vomition repetitive urination and defecation, aimless running and barking. tenesmus, dyspnoea and tonic-cloric seizures sign in advanced stage. Horses (mainly heart affected): Cardiac arrest and sudden death.
Strychnine	Nervous	Nervousness, restlessness, excitement, muscular twitching, dilated pupils, hyperthermia and neck stiffness lead to ophisthotonus (saw horse). Death occurs due to spasms of the respiratory muscles or paralysis of the respiratory center.
Warfarin and Congeners	Coagulative mechanism of blood	Massive internal and external hemorrhages, blood oozing from body orifices, visible haematomas under skin and around joints, purpura, dyspnoea, weakness and shock. Clinical signs may depend on site haemorrhage.
Alphanaphthyl-thiourea (ANTU)	Gastrointestinal, respiratory	Vomiting, salivation, respiratory distress, cyanosis, pulmonary oedema and white foamy discharged from the nostrils and the oral cavity lead to asphyxia, coma and deaths.

Fungicide Toxicity

Fungicide	*Major Body System/ Organs Affected*	*Symptoms*
Pentachloro-phenol (PCP)	Nervous and dermal	Nervousness, increase pulse and respiratory rate, weakness, muscle tremors, anorexia, hyperthermia, convulsions and death. Skin contact develops hyperkeratosis, erythema, dermatitis and acne. Chronic: emaciation, fever, anemia, abortions, still birth, foetal malformations in pregnant animals.

Mycotoxine Toxicity

Mycotoxine	*Major Body System/ Organs Affected*	*Symptoms*
Aflatoxins	Bone, liver, immune, gastrointestinal	Acute: Anorexia, vomiting, depression, dyspnoea, coughing, nasal discharge, hemorrhage (epistaxis and bloody faeces), anaemia, in appetence and death. Sub acute: weakness, reduced growth and feed efficiency, jaundice, haematomas, haemorrhagic enteritis (warfarin like condition) and death.In cattle, there may be blindness, moving in circles, ear twitching, teeth grinding, photosensitive dermatitis, ataxia etc. Chronic: Off feed, weight loss, rough hair coat, anaemia, enlarged abdomen, mild jaundice, depression and anorexia. Poultry: Reduce in weight gain, feed intake, feed conversion efficiency, fertility and hatchability.
Ergot	Nervous, circulatory	Nervous form: Anorexia, lameness (hind limb affected first), swelling and tenderness of the fetlock joint and pastern hyperthermia and hyper salivation. Gangrenous form: Necrosis of the ear, tail, feet and hind quarter. Sloughing off claws, hooves and tail. No udder development and agalactia in late pregnancy of swine, cattle, and horses.
Ochratoxins	Gastrointestinal, immune, liver, kidney	Weight loss, reduced feed intake, polyuria, polydypsia and dehydration, immunosuppression, teratogenicity, carcinogenicity.

Plant Toxicity

Plant Toxin	*Major Body System/ Organs Affected*	*Symptoms*
Cyanogenetic Plants (sorghum, Sudan grass)	Respiratory, blood	Per acute or acute: Laboured and quick breathing, stumbling gait, and dyspnoea, bright red gum, eye sclera, and mucous membranes, excessive salivation and lacrimation and death within few hours.
Sweet pea (*Lathyrus odoratus*)	Bone	Cattle: Osteolathyrism, lameness, pain in the feet and disinclination to rise. Horse: Osteolathyrism (long bone curvature, kyphosis, scoliosis, osteoporosis, and poor development of connective tissue).
Bracken fern	Gastrointestinal, nervous	Ruminants: Dermatitis, anaemia, petechial haemorrhages, haematochezia, bright blindness and haematuria due to urinary tumours (enzootic haematuria). Horse: Thiamine deficiency (braken staggers) include anorexia, incordination and staggering gait. Animals stand with feet well spread and back arched clonic spasms and death. Pigs: anorexia, weight loss terminal recumbency, dyspnoeaa and death.
Oxalate poisoning	Gastrointestinal, respiratory, nervous	Acute: Dullness, lowering of the head, loss of appetite, stasis of rumen motility, bloat, salivation, progressive weakness, laboured respiration, dilatation of pupils, twitching of muscles, tetany, convulsions and death mainly due to shock. Subacute: Stiff gait, frequent urination, red brown colour urine, recumbency. Chronic: Uremia.
Lantana camara		Antimuscaranic effect (Similar to atropine effect) Dryness of mouth and throat, dysphagia and difficulty in swallowing, photophobia, dilated pupils, urine incontinent respiratory failure and death.
Datura	Anticholinergic	Dryness mouth and throat, dysphagia, staggering gait, photophobia, dilated pupils, inco-ordination, inability to pass urine. Death may occur from respiratory failure.

Animal Poisoning

Animal Toxin	*Major Body System/ Organs Affected*	*Symptoms*
Snakes	Circulatory, nervous	Pit viper (rattlesnakes): Marked swelling and discolouration of the tissues and dark bloody fluid may ooze from bite site, hypothermia, dilated pupils and complete unconsciousness. Extensive local suppuration, sloughing and gangrene, and malignant oedema or tetanus may supervene or death may occur from septicaemia. Krait: Violent abdominal pain and convulsions may precede death. In calves, the effects of the neurotoxin are manifested by marked papillary dilatations, excitement, incoordination and later paralysis. Elapine snakebites: Systemic neurological signs predominate. *i.e* muscular weakness developing into paralysis.
Scorpions	Circulatory	Profuse and sometimes frothy salivation, vigorous head shaking, pawing at the mouth and retching. With more severe intoxication, cardiac arrhythmias, dyspnoea, cyanosis and convulsions are produced. Ventricular fibrillation precedes death heart failure.

Drugs Poisoning

Drugs Toxin	*Major Body System/ Organs Affected*	*Symptoms*
Phenothiazine	Blood	Horses: Haemolysis of erythrocytes includes icterus, anaemia and haemoglobinuria. Ruminants: Photosensitization signs
Salicylates	Gastrointestinal, respiratory	Haematemesis and gastric irritation or ulceration, respiratory alkalosis, metabolic acidosis, stillbirths, lethargy, hyperpnoea, increased blood coagulation time.
Digitalis	Gastrointestinal, cardiac, nervous	In appetence, vomiting, diarrhoea, blurred vision, contracted pupils, dizziness, excessive urination, cardiac arrhythmia atrioventricular block and nervous disturbances.
Chlorpromazine	Nervous	Incoordination and excitement in horses, violent reaction alternates with periods of sedation. Chronic case show jaundice, drowsiness, dizzness, fatigue, dryness of mouth, urinary retention and constipation

Self Assessment

Fill in the Blank

1. ________ is blood plasma without fibrinogen or the other clotting factors
2. For routine hematology anticoagulant EDTA is used ________.mg/10 ml blood.
3. In rat blood is collected from ________. and ________.
4. For preservation of synovial fluid preservative used is________
5. Insulin secreted from ________. Cells of pancreas and regulate ________.
6. Write two main cause of KETOSIS in animals

   1. ________.2________
7. Write name of 3 main type of Diabetes mellatus.

   1________.2________3________
8. Write name of Ketone bodies

   1________2________.3________
9. In E.C.F primary anioin is________
10. Creatinine test is more specific for ________.dysfunction
11. In pig blood is collected from ________. and ________.
12. For preservation of urine preservative used is________ and ________.
13. Write two main cause of protein deficiency in animals

    1.________. 2________

14. In E.C.F primary cation is________

15. To obtain cell free plasma anticoagulated blood centrifuge at ________. rpm for ________.min.

16. In rabbit blood is collected from ________. and ________.

17. Glucagon hormone secreted from ________. Cells of pancreas.

18. Normally the ratio of albumin and globulin is ________

19. When separating serum or plasma, the temperature should not be below ________.

20. Write name of ketone bodies

    1. ________. 2. ________ 3. ________

21. Cause of pre renal azotemia is

    1. ________. 2. ________.

22. Antibiogram drug sensitivity by disc diffusion method is done in ________media.

23. Two most important name of enzyme used in liver function test are________ and ________

24. Substrate used in ELISA is ________.

25. Conjugate used in ELISA is ________.

26. ________ g bone is required for toxicological examination.

27. Antidote of copper is________.

28. Nalorphine is antidote of ________.

29. Unconjugate Bilirubin is react with ________. to form Conjugate bilirubin.

30. Porphyrin ring of hemoglobin breaks in ________, ________ and ________.

31. Deficiency of.. is easily revealed by means of a film strip test and gelatin test.

32. For toxicological the quantity of hair required________.g.

33. For toxicological the quantity of blood required________.ml

34. Antidote of lead is________.

35. **Antidote of Nitrite, nitrate, chlorate is________**

36. **Antidote of opiates is________.**

37. **Benidict test is used for detection of ________ is urine sample.**

38. **In urine sample test used for detection of bile pigment________.**

39. **PCV is done in ________. Tube.**

40. **For making blood smear methanol is used for________**

41. **Increased total erythrocyte countcorresponding increase in Hb and PCV is k/a________**

42. **Normocytic and normochromic RBC is seen in ________.**

43. **Normal range of Hb in cattle is________.**

44. **In direct wet mount faecal examination slide is seen at________.X objective lens.**

45. **$ZnSO_4$ (33 per cent) solution is used in faecal examination in ________ method.**

46. **EPG is method of ________.estimation of parasites in faecal examination.**

47. **If blood is present in faeces it is termed as________.**

48. **Needle of ________ gauge is used for blood collection in poultry.**

49. **Monocytic leukemia mostly occurs in ________.**

50. **Blood agar is a ________. Media.**

Tick the most Appropriate Answer

1. **Polyuria is found in case of**
   a. Fever
   b. Shock
   c. Diabetes mellitus
   d. All of the above

2. **Red urine is found in**
   a. Hemoglobin (blood, free)
   b. Myoglobin
   c. Porphyrian
   d. All of the above

3. **Protein test in urine is done by**
   a. Sulphosalicylic acid test
   b. Heller's ring test
   c. Sulpher test
   d. Both a and b

4. Gmelin test is done for

a. Bile pigment b. Protein
c. Glucose d. Blood

5. Wintrobe tube is primerly used for the estimation of

a. DLC b. Hb
c. TLC d. PCV

6. Fecal examination is indicated in .... conditions.

a. Eosinophilia b. Anemia
c. Icterus d. all

7. The larvae are separated from faecal culture by _______ method.

a. Zeil- Neelson b. Baerman
c. Gorcotts d. None of above

8. Canine has more _______ than lymphocytes

a. Monocytes b. Eosinophils
c. Neutrophils d. Basophils

9. pH of normal milk is

a. 6.5 b. 7.5
c. 5.5 d. 8.5

10. Tissue should be collected directly in to _______ for histopathology

a. Water b. Ice
c. Fixative d. None

11. Haemoglobulineria occurs in

a. Leptospirosis b. Pasteurellosis
c. Tuberculosis d. Brucellosis

12. Type II diabetes mellatus is

a. Juvinile diabetes b. Adult on-set diabetes
c. Genetic diabetes d. Gestational diabetes

13. In pre-renal azotemia kidney will be

a. Highly affected b. Moderate affected
c. Normal in function d. None

14. $CuSO_4$ is used in the staining of

a. Cell membrane b. Capsule
c. Spore d. Flagella

15. BUN and Creatinine is measured for the diagnosis of abnormal function of

a. Liver
b. Pancreas
c. Kidney
d. Heart

16. Antidote of nitrate, nitrite and chlorate is

a. Methylene blue
b. BAL
c. Deferoxamine
d. Tannic acid

17. The process of exclusion in closely related disease is known as

a. Test therapy diagnosis
b. Clinical diagnosis
c. Laboratory diagnosis
d. Differential diagnosis

18. Increased TLC is referred to as_______

a. Leucopenia
b. Leucocytosis
c. Leukemia
d. Lymphocytosis

19. The TLC count 6000/cu mm of blood will be_______ per liter blood

a. 6 10^9
b. 6 10^6
c. 6 10^3
d. 6 101^2

20. If no parasitic ova are detected in direct smear method saturate the sample should be declaired_______

a. Negative
b. Positive
c. For re-examination by flotation
d. None of the above

21. To preserve the faecal sample, _______ is added as preservative.

a. 10 per cent ethanol
b. 10 per cent formalin
c. 10 per cent methanol
d. 10 per cent acetone

22. Teats should be washed with _______before collection of milk samples for the laboratory examination.

a. 70 per cent ethanol
b. 70 per cent formalin
c. Per cent acetone
d. None of the above

23. Washing solution in ELISA is _______

a. PBS
b. Tris buffer
c. PBS-Tween
d. PBS- conjugate

24. Strychnine can be detected in

a. Stomach content
b. Liver
c. Urine
d. All of the above

25. Whole blood minus both the cells and clotting factor is k/a

a. PCV
b. Plasma
c. Serum
d. Hb

26. Advantage of anticoagulant is

a. Least effect on size and haemolysis of RBC
b. Used for blood transfusion
c. For routine haematology
d. All of the above

27. In dog blood is collected from

a. Jugular vein
b. Ear vein
c. Cephalic vein
d. Wing vein

28. Type II diabetes mellatus is

a. Juvenile diabetes
b. Adult on-set diabetes
c. Genetic diabetes
d. All of the above

29. Glucagon harmone is secreted by

a. Liver
b. Kidney
c. Pancreas
d. Spleen

30. Elivated serum conc. of triglyceride is due to

a. Hypothyroidism
b. D.M
c. Anaemia
d. Both a and b

31. Role of Ca in body is

a. Skeleton formation
b. Enzyme activation
c. Blood cogulation
d. All of the above

32. In pre-renal azotemia kidney will be

a. Highly affected
b. Moderate affected
c. Normal in function
d. Least affected

33. Sweetish or fruity odour in urine indicate presence of

a. Glucose
b. Ketone bodies
c. Blood
d. Urea

34. In urine sample Sulphosalicylic test is used for detection of

a. Glucose
b. Protein
c. Bile salt
d. Urea

35. Majority of the parasites/ectoparasite are

a. Leeches and ticks
b. Monogenetic trematodes
c. Mange- mites
d. Arthopodes

36. Macrocytes are typically seen in ________ deficiency.

a. Folic acid
b. Vitamin B_{12}
c. Both a and b
d. None

37. Morbid changes are

a. Alterations found in tissue at necropsy
b. Alterations found in tissue at biopsy
c. Alterations found in tissue as symptom
d. None of the above

38. P.M. examination in vet. medicine known as

a. Necropsy
b. Autopsy
c. Biopsy
d. Any of above

39. Main components of blood clot is

a. Fibrin
b. R.B.C.
c. platelet
d. All of the above

40. Presence of cast of urine is known as

a. Bilirubinuria
b. Globulinuria
c. Proteinuria
d. Cylindruria

41. EDTA is an antidote for which of the following

a. Sodium secobarbital
b. Asprin
c. Phosphorus
d. Lead

42. Techoic acid is present in the cell wall of

a. Gram positive
b. Gam negative
c. Both and b
d. None of the above

43. Bacteria which remain red coloured after ZN staining are

a. Acid fast bacteria
b. Partial acid fast bacteria
c. Non acid fast bacteria
d. Gram variable bacteria

44. In staphylococcus infection partial haemolysis is on the basis of

a. Coagulation test
b. Dick test
c. CAMP test
d. None of the above

45. Medium which is suitable for the growth of a specific organism is termed as

a. Selective media
b. Minimal media
c. Complete media
d. None of the above

46. *Taenia saginata* is pathogenic to

a. Dog
b. Cat
c. Man
d. Pig

47. Normally eggs are operculated in

a. Trematode
b. Roundworm
c. Noth
d. None of the above

48. fasciola hepatica present in

a. Liver
b. Caecum
c. Small intestine
d. None of the above

49. Erythrocytes arranged in a roll is called

a. Rouleaux
b. Ovalocyte
c. Band cell
d. Shift to left

50. Thickness of blood smear depends upon

a. Size of drop
b. Angle of spreader
c. Both a and b
d. None of the above

Match the Following

A.

1.	Haemocytometer method	a	egg count technique
2.	TLC	b.	Methanol
3.	Basophilic cells	c.	larvae of certain parasites
4.	Giemsa	d.	Flotation technique
5.	Nucleated RBCs	e.	centrifugal flotation
6.	Saturated sugar solution	f.	20
7.	Lane's method	g.	Bird
8.	Baermann's Technique	h.	Inflammation
9.	Stoll's dilution	i	TEC
10.	mite infestation	j	10 per cent NaOH or KOH

B

1.	Willi's method	a	Methanol
2.	eosinophilic cells	b.	Flotation technique
3.	Giemsa	c.	TRP
4.	Nucleated RBCs	d.	Parasitic infection
5.	Dog (Hb)	e.	12-18 (g/dl)
6.	Skin scrapping	f.	10 per cent NaOH or KOH
7.	Neutrophilia shift to left	g.	Biopsy
8.	Interventional cytology	h.	Bird
9.	Calcium	i.	BUN X 2.14
10.	Urea	j.	blood coagulation

C

1.	Elevated level of lipase	a.	Crystal violet
2.	α- cells	b.	biopsy
3.	Arginine	c.	Acute pancreatic necrosis
4.	Histopathology	d.	paraffin wax
5.	Fixation	e.	Indole test
6.	Impregnation	f.	pathological alternations in tissue
7.	Cytology	g.	Ziehl- Neilson's staining
8.	Primary stain	h.	Liver
9.	Mycobacterium	i.	Glucagon
10.	Kovác's reagent	j.	Buffer formalin

D

1.	Gram staining counter stain	a.	Trepnema
2.	Viral specimen	b.	Actinobacillus
3.	acid fast staining	c.	Drug sensitivity
4.	Spiral like cork screw	d.	HRP
5.	Short coccoid rods	e.	quantative
6.	Modified Kirby-Beaur method	f.	safranin or dilute carbol fuschin
7.	H_2S positive, indole negative	g.	H_2O_2
8.	ELISA conjugate	h.	Methylene blue
9.	Substrate	i.	Salmonella
10.	Tube agglutination	j.	Penicillin and Streptomycin

E.

1.	Viral sample	a.	Safranine
2.	Bacteriological sample	b.	sarcine
3.	Histopathological examination	c.	proteus
4.	Parasitological examination	d.	70 per cent alcohol
5.	Anaerobic media	e.	Kept at 4°C
6.	Mycological sample	f.	RCM
7.	Gram's counter stain	g.	$CuSO_4$ (20 per cent)
8.	Capsule staining	h.	50 per cent buffer glycerine sol.
9.	Gram possitive cocci of eight	i	SDA
10.	Swarming phenomenon	j	10 per cent formaline

Write True/False

1. Heparin-Least effect on size and haemolysis of RBCs.
2. In rat site of blood collection is Cardiac (anesthetized only), marginal ear vein.
3. 10 per cent Formalin is used for the preservative of faeces.
4. A decrease in serum total proteins may results from heavy losses of proteins in urine as in nephritic syndrome.
5. An elevated level of serum triglycerides decreases blood viscosity.
6. Creatinine is produced due of metabolism of lipid.
7. Gmelin test is done for bile salt.
8. Thymol is used for the preservative of faeces.
9. Saturated sugar solution is used in flotation method for detection of parasitic eggs.
10. LDL (low density lipid) is known bad cholesterol.
11. Sulphur powder is used for detection of protein in urine.
12. Wintrobe tube is used for packed cell volume.
13. ESR (Erythrocyte sedimentation rate) of Dog and cat is 1 hour.
14. In Leishman staining smear is fixed in methanol for 3 min.
15. Methyl red test is used to determine whether the some bacteria perform mixed acid fermentation when supplied glucose.
16. Modified Kirby-Beaur method is used to study drug sensitivity by dilution method.

17. Agar gel precipitation test is quantitative method to detect the presence of antigen in sample or antibody in serum.
18. ELISAs can provide a useful measurement of only antigen concentration.
19. PBS Tween is used as blocking solution in ELISA procedure.
20. Poisoning of lead affects nervous and bone mainly.
21. Carbamate and Organochlorine is insecticide poison.
22. Pancreas is a gland or organ in the digestive and endocrine system of vertebrates.
23. Range of blood glucose in cattle is 60-100 mg/dl.
24. β cells of islets of Langerhans of pancreas secrete insulin.
25. Antidote of iron is EDTA.
26. Required serum quantity for toxicological exam is 5 ml.
27. Bromothymol blue test is done for milk test.
28. Neubaur chamber ids used for quantative faecal test.
29. If blood is present in urine called Haematuria.
30. Triglycerides are complexes with cholesterol, phospholipids and plasma proteins to form lipoproteins.
31. Females of any species are less susceptible to ketosis than corresponding males.
32. Benedict reagent is used for protein test in urine.
33. Wet mount faecal examination is done at 40 x in microscope.
34. Range of haemoglobin in dog is 10 -13 g/dl.
35. Antibiogram drug sensitivity by disc diffusion method is done in Muller Hilton media.
36. Tube agglutination test is quantative test.
37. Slide agglutination test is a quantitative test.
38. Milk ring test is used in anthrax test.
39. Substrate used in ELISA is H_2O_2.
40. Conjugate used in ELISA is Horse Reddish Peroxidase.
41. 250 g bone is required for toxicological examination.
42. Nalorphine is antidote of cyanide.
43. Antidote of copper is Mo.

44. Red colour urine is seen in haemoglobinuria, myoglobinuria and drugs used like phenolphthalein.
45. Level of glucose in urine increases in diabetic ketosis and starvation.
46. Hay test is used for detection of bile salts in urine.
47. Erythrocytes related tests are Hb, PCV and TEC.
48. Quantity of liver and spleen required for toxicological examination is 3000 g.
49. In fowl normal value of haemoglobin is 8.83-11.3 g/gl.
50. Babesia and Theileria is intracellular haemoprotozoan.

Answers Key

Fill in the Blank

1. Blood serum
2. 10-20
3. Retro-orbital plexus, cardiac puncture
4. 3.8 per cent sodium citrate
5. β- cells of island of Langerhans, blood glucose
6. Diabetes mellitus, starvation.
7. Insulin dependent diabetes mellitus, non insulin dependent diabetes mellitus and gestational diabetes mellitus
8. Acetone, Acetoacetic acid and β-hydrobutyric acid
9. Chloride ion
10. Renal
11. Ear vein and anterior venacava
12. Thymol and formalin
13. Nephritic syndrome and intestinal malabsorption
14. Sodium ion
15. 2000 to 3000g for 15 min
16. Cardiac (anesthetized only), marginal ear vein
17. α cells
18. 2:1
19. 15°C
20. Obstruction in urater, Neoplasia
21. Reduced cardiac output, Shock
22. Muller Hilton
23. Serum Glutamic Pyruvic Transaminase and Serum Glutamic Oxaloacetic transaminase
24. Hydrogen per oxide
25. Horse reddish per oxidase
26. 250

27. Penicillamine molybdenum salts
28. Opiates
29. Glucuronic acid
30. Biliverdin, iron and globin
31. Faecal trypsin
32. 5.0
33. 10-30
34. BAL (British Antilewisite or dimercaprol), calcium disodium EDTA
35. Methylene blue
36. Nalorphine
37. Glucose
38. Gmelin test
39. Wintribe
40. Fixation
41. Polycythemia
42. Anaemia, Inherited enzyme deficiency, acute haemorrhage
43. 8-14(11) g/dl
44. 10
45. Flotation method
46. Qualitative
47. Melena
48. 20
49. Cat
50. Enriched

Tick the Most Appropriate Answer

1.	c	2.	d	3.	d	4.	a	5.	d
6.	d	7.	b	8.	c	9.	a	10.	c
11.	a	12.	b	13.	c	14.	b	15.	c
16.	a	17.	d	18.	b	19.	a	20.	c
21.	b	22.	a	23.	c	24.	d	25.	c
26.	d	27.	c	28.	b	29.	c	30.	d
31.	d	32.	c	33.	b	34.	b	35.	d
36.	c	37.	a	38.	a	39.	a	40.	c
41.	d	42.	a	43.	a	44.	c	45.	a
46.	c	47.	a	48.	a	49.	a	50.	b

Match the Following

A.

1. i 2. f 3. h 4. b 5. g 6. d 7. e 8. c 9. a 10. j

B.

1. b 2. d 3. a 4. h 5. e 6. f 7. c 8. g 9. j 10. i

C.

1. c 2. i 3. h 4. f 5. j 6. d 7. b 8. a 9. g 10. e

D.

1. f 2. h 3. b 4. a 5. b 6. c 7. i 8. a 9. g 10. e

E.

1. h 2. e 3. j 4. d 5. f 6. i 7. a 8. g 9. a 10. c

Write True/False

1.	True	2.	False	3.	True	4.	True	5.	False
6.	False	7.	False	8.	False	9.	True	10.	True
11.	False	12.	True	13.	True	14.	False	15.	True
16.	True	17.	False	18.	False	19.	False	20.	False
21.	True	22.	True	23.	False	24.	True	25.	False
26.	False	27.	True	28.	False	29.	True	30.	True
31.	False	32.	False	33.	False	34.	False	35.	True
36.	True	37.	False	38.	False	39.	True	40.	True
41.	True	42.	False	43.	True	44.	True	45.	False
46.	True	47.	True	48.	False	49.	True	50.	True

Appendix

Reagent/Solution

1. Diazo Reagent

Stock solution (A)	
Sulphanilic acid	1.0 g
Distilled water	200 ml
Conc. hydrochloric acid	1.0 ml
Stock solution (B)	
sodium nitrite	0.5 g
Distilled water	100 ml
Working reagent (C)	
Stock solution (A)	10 ml mix well before use
Stock solution (B)	0.1 ml

2. RBC Diluting Fluid

a. Gower's solution	
Sodium sulphate	2.5 g
Glacial acetic acid	16.6 ml
Distilled water	100.0 ml
b. Hayem's fluid	
Sodium sulphate	2.5 g
Sodium chloride	0.5 g
Mercuric chloride	0.5 g
Distilled water	100.0 ml

3. WBC Diluting Fluid

a. For animals:

Glacial acetic acid	3.0 ml
Distilled water	97.0 ml

Add few drops of aqueous methylene blue to give colour to the solution

b. For birds:

Sodium citrate	3.8 g
Formalin (neutral)	0.2 ml
Brilliant cresyl blue	0.5 g
Distilled water	100.0 ml

4. Benedicts Reagent

Solution (a)

Sodium carbonate	100.0 ml
Distilled water	800.0 ml

Dissolve by heating

Sodium citrate	200.0 g
Potassium thiocyanate	125.0 g

Mix well and dissolve

Solution (b)

Copper sulphate	18.0 g
Distilled water	100.0 ml

Dissolve by shaking

Solution (c)

Potassium ferrocyanide	0.25 g
Distilled water	5 ml

Dissolve by shaking

Mix the solution a, b and c at room temperature and make up the volume to 1000 ml with distilled water. Keep the solution in a dark coloured bottle.

5. Robert's Reagent

Solution (a)

Magnesium sulfate saturated solution in distilled water

Solution (b)

Concentrated nitric acid

Working reagent

Solution (a)	5 parts
Solution (b)	1 parts

6. Sodium Nitroprusside Solutions

Sodium nitroprusside	10.0 g
Distilled water	20.0 ml

Dissolve by heating

7. Biuret Reagent

(Benidicts qualitative reagent)

Solution (a)

Cupric sulphate pentahydrate	17.3 g
Distilled water	100.0 ml

Solution (b)

Sodium citrate	173.0 g
Sodium carbonate	100.0 g
Distilled water	800.0 ml

Dissolve by heating mix solution (a) and solution (b) and make it 1000 ml by distill water.

8. EDTA Solution

Tetra sodium EDTA	5.0 g
Distilled water	100.0 ml

9. Urease Solution

Glycerin	67.0 ml
Distilled water	33 ml
Urease	2.0 g

10. Zinc Sulphate Solution

Zinc sulphate	50.0 g
Distilled water	1000.0 ml

11. Iodine Solution

Iodine crystals	2.0 g
Potassium iodide	3.0 g
Distilled water	100.0 ml

12. Nessler's Solution

Potassium iodide	30.0 g
Iodine crystals	22.5 g
Distilled water	20.0 ml

Mix to dissolve. Add metallic mercury 30.0 g. Dilute to 200 ml with distilled water and mix it with 975 ml of 10 per cent NaOH

13. Normal Saline Solution

Sodium chloride	0.85 g
Distilled water	100.0 ml

14. Phosphate Buffer Saline (PBS) (pH 7.2)

Sodium chloride	8.0 g
Potassium chloride	0.20 g
Potassium dihydrogen orthophosphate	0.20 g
Disodium hydrogen orthophosphate	2.312 g
Distilled water	1000.0 ml

15. Lugol's Iodine

Iodine crystal	1.0 g
Potassium iodide	2.0 g
Distilled water	100.0 g

16. Kovac's Reagent

Amyl alcohol	75 ml
Para dimethyl amino benzaldehyde	5.0 g
Conc. Hydrochloric acid	25 ml

17. Methyl Red Reagent

Methyl red	0.02 g
95 per cent ethanol	100.0 ml

18. Formal Saline

35-40 per cent formaldehyde	10.0 ml
Normal saline solution	100.0 ml

19. Buffered Formalin

35-40 per cent formaldehyde	10.0 ml
PBS (pH 7.2)	100.0 ml

20. Phosphate Buffer (pH 7.2)

Solution (a)	
Na_2HPO_4	35.61 g
Distilled water	100.0 ml
Solution (b)	
Na_2HPO_4	27.67 g
Distilled water	1000.0 ml
Solution (a)	28.0 ml
Solution (b)	72.0 ml
Distilled water to	200.0 ml

21. Coating Buffer (pH 9.6)

Sodium carbonate (Na_2CO_3)	1.59 g
Sodium bicarbonate ($NaHCO_3$)	2.93 g
Distilled water to	1000.0 ml

22. Washing Solution (pH 7.2)

Sodium chloride	20.20 g
Potassium dihydrogen phosphate (KH_2PO_4)	2.0 g
Disodium hydrogen phosphate ($Na_2HPO_42H_2O$)	1.15 g
Tween- 20	0.5 ml
Distilled water to	1000.0 ml

23. Ringer's Solution

Solution chloride	0.7 g
Potassium chloride	0.026 g
Sodium bicarbonate	0.03 g
Calcium chloride	0.003 g
Distilled water	1000.0 ml

24. Methylene Blue Stain

Methylene blue	0.03 g
95 per cent ethanol	30.0 ml
Distilled water to	100.0 ml

25. Giemsa Stain

Stock solution	
Azure II- eosin	3.0 g
Azure II	0.8 g
Glycerol	250 ml
Acetone free methanol	250 ml
Working stain: stock solution	1 part
Distilled water	9 part

26. Leishman's Stain

Leishman's stain powder	0.15 g
Methanol	100.0 ml

Mix in pestle and mortar. Filter before use

27. Lactophenol Cotton Blue Stain

Phenol crystal	10 g
Lactic acid syrup	10 ml
Glycerol	20 ml
Distilled water to	10 ml
Cotton blue stain/aniline blue	50 mg

28. Gram's Staining (smears)

a. *Stock solution A: 1 per cent crystal violet in ethanol*

Stock solution B: 1 per cent ammonium oxalate

Working solution:

Stock solution A	20 ml
Stock solution B	80 ml

b. *Gram's iodine*

Iodine crystals	1.0 g
Potassium iodide	2.0 g
Distilled water	300 ml

c. *Decolorizer*

Ethanol (95 per cent)	250 ml
Acetone	250 ml

d. *Counter stain*

Safranin	2.5 g
95 per cent ethanol	100 ml

Working stain: safranin1:4 diluted with distilled water

29. Harris Haematoxylene

Haematoxylene	2.5 g
Absolute ethanol	50 ml
Potassium alum	50 g
Distilled water	500 ml
Mercuric oxide	1.5 g
Glacial acetic acid	20 ml

Filter before use

30. Mayer's Haematoxylene

Haematoxylene	0.5 g
Distilled water	500 ml
Potassium alum	25 g
Sodium iodide	0.1 g

Citric acid	0.5 g
Chloral hydrate	25.0 g

31. Acid Alcohol

Conc. HCl	3.0 ml
70 per cent ethanol	97.0 ml

32. Eosin

a. Aqueous: eosin	1.0 g	
Distilled water		100 ml
b. Alcoholic: eosin	1.0 g	
70 per cent ethanol		100 ml

33. Periodic Acid-Schiff's Staining

a. Periodic acid

Periodic acid	0.4 g
Distilled water	10.0 ml
2.72 per cent sodium acetate solution	5.0 ml
Ethanol	35.0 ml

b. Reducing sugar

Potassium iodide	1.0 g
Sodium thiosulphate	1.0 g
Distilled water	20 ml
Ethanol	30 ml
1N HCl	1.0 ml

c. Schiff's reagent

Basic fuchsin	1.0 g
Distilled water	200 ml

Boil and cool to 50°C, filter; add 20 ml 1N HCl, cool to 25°C and add sodium metabisulfite 1.0 g, store for 24 hours in dark and add 2.0 g activated charcoal. Shake, filter and keep in dark in stoppered bottle at 4°C

34. Nutrient Broth

Beef extract	0.3 g
Peptone	0.5 g
Distilled water	100.0 ml

35. Nutrient Agar

Nutrient broth	100 ml
Agar	1.5 g

Sterilize by autoclave

36. Simmon's Citrate Agar

Sodium chloride	2.5 g
Sodium citrate	1.0 g
Magnesium sulphate	0.1 g
Monoammonium phosphate	0.5 g
Di potassium phosphate	0.5 g
Bacto- agar	7.5 g
Distilled water	500 ml

pH 6.8 autoclave at 121°C for 15 min.

37. Sabouraud's Dextrose Agar

Peptone	1.0 g
Dextrose	40.0 g
Agar	18.0 g
Distilled water	1000.0 ml

pH 5.6 autoclave at 121°C for 15 min.